Your Health Turned On

Empowering Women to turn off:
disease. obesity. dieting

Kat Wright ND
Traditional Naturopath ND

First Edition December 2010

Your Health Turned On

Empowering women to turn off: obesity.diabeties.dieting

Kat Wright ND

This is a workbook to follow up on the commitment made to pursue a life of health and wellness in body, mind and spirit for the benefit of all you contact on your journey!

ISBN: 1-4564-7752-8
ISBN-13: 9781456477523

ACKNOWLEDGMENTS

I thank my God for the enormous opportunities provided to me, and my family and friends who, over the years, have encouraged me by taking care of their health and personal growth.

The YMCA for being a body/mind/spirit organization visibly committed to community.

I also want to thank the leaders in the alternative health community, who, by their hard work and commitment to change, have forged the way and set the path for anyone who wants to come after.

I thank Alternative Medical Doctors, Chiropractors, Naturopaths, Massage Therapists, Herbalists, Iridologists, Health Food Store Owners, Certified Natural Health Professionals and Alternative Health Educators, who have been willing to work together to educate and promote wellness on all levels. It has been an uphill battle without much recognition by a committed few.

NOTE TO THE READER

Your Health Turned On is based on personal observation, experience and study of over thirty years.

The information in this book is not intended as a replacement for professional medical care or advice, nor to endorse or recommend any particular product or company.

If you take medication or have a medically related issue, I encourage you to always seek professional medical help before making lifestyle changes.

ENDORSEMENTS

DR JODY VAN JURA As a family medicine physician I was trained to treat illnesses and diseases, with little focus on prevention. Over the last 10 years I have grown to appreciate looking more at the preventative aspects of medicine both in the pediatric and adult population. Personally and professionally I have a passion for healthy living, both with diet and exercise. *Your Health Turned On* is a book in which most of my patients including myself can read to be motivated to carry out this lifestyle. It is not a question of "if" but "when" we should all adopt these healthy habits in order to live a quality life. Medicines should be used to augment healthy living to treat common disorders such as diabetes, hypertension, coronary artery disease, etc., not to act in replacement for living well. I feel that if most individuals would read and live by even 50% of the principles addressed in this book we would not even have to debate a fix to our healthcare system as costs would dramatically go down and quality of life would rise. Prevention is the key to healthy living.

Jodi Van Jura, M.D. Springboro Ohio

Board Certified in Family Medicine
Full Time outpatient practice
Medical Director for KMC Community Wellness
Medical Advisory Board Member for The Miami Valley Women's Center

DR CAROL LOCKENGER Kathy has given a wonderful guide for all women to teach them how to be responsible for their own health. Women are the great influence of the family and it is women who can change and transform the health of the family, which will benefit future generations. This book is a great source of information and guidance for women because they hold the key to health in their hands.

Carol M. Loechinger, D.C., N.M.D.
CHIROPRACTIC & NATUROPATHIC PHYSICIAN

DR GREARD POORTINGA You may have been attracted by Kathy's sparkle, but her advice is based on a depth of experience. In the decades I have known Kathy she has worked to help numerous individuals improve their lives, from teaching macrobiotic cooking to cancer sufferers to helping teenage swimmers improve their performance. Her knowledge is not based just on her study, but also on years of coaching real people to find solutions that really work. Kathy's passion for changing health care is expressed by her commitment to helping you.

Gerard Poortinga, DC, FIAMA, DACAN
Applied Kinesiology and Clinical Nutrition

TINA WOODS My husband was diagnosed with prostate cancer and was scheduled for a radical prostatectomy when we started talking to Kathy about the role of the body in recovery. Kathy's supportive approaches were a much valued help towards his recovery.

After reading *Your Health Turned On* we researched the issues further and felt that eating healthier was valuable for our entire family. We started on a nutrient dense plant based diet and discarded the toxic Standard American Diet (SAD) that we had followed for the past forty years.

After just three months of adding raw juices and healthy recipes, my husband's health and my health had drastically improved; we both felt better than we had in years, in spite of the cancer. We saw major improvement in the behavior and health of our children as well. Our young sons displayed more control and focus at school and swimming and had less allergy problems. While the kids are not vegans, they no longer eat foods that are loaded with nitrates and eat mostly organic meats. Since starting our new diets I am convinced that healthy eating is a key factor in the prevention and mitigation of serious disease. Most people do not understand the harm the SAD diet is causing them and have a great misconception about how the foods they eat are affecting their health.

We never want to go back to our previous lifestyle, and wish everyone would change their habits to prevent cancer and other degenerative disease. Thank you Kathy!

Tina Woods/Attorney
Dayton, Ohio

Do not believe in anything simply because you have heard it.

Do not believe in anything simply because it is spoken and rumored by many.

Do not believe in anything simply because it is found written in your religious books.

Do not believe in anything merely on the authority of your teachers and elders.

Do not believe in traditions because they have been handed down for many generations.

But after observation and analysis, when you find that anything agrees with reason and is conducive to the good and benefit of one and all, then accept it and live up to it.

     - Buddha

CONTENTS

it is so hard when I have to and so easy when I want to
       - Annie Gottlier

PREFACE

Your Health Turned On is about thinking and choices; about how they affect your health as well as the health of those around you. I will help you cut through the confusion in the media and magazines today. You will get strategies to grow towards lifelong health and understand it is possible to live a life without disease.

Many, possibly most, will come to this work because of a diagnosis. I am praying you will pass this on to those still with time and health-before the diagnosis. Everything in this book can help a healing body. You alone are responsible for your choices, but how can you choose without knowledge. I am giving you knowledge. I have helped many find the answers they needed to heal their disease. I have helped many prevent disease; these are the rare who are motivated towards good and not away from pain. Will you wait until your diagnosis? Will you become one of the statistics? I am praying not.

This is about empowerment. You are empowered to accomplish whatever it is you desire by following these simple ideas. You must renew your mind or change the way you think if you want to change anything in your life. Old habits and belief systems that do not create health and are not serving you can be changed.

My experience with people who have chosen to take personal responsibility and pursue their dreams has proven to me that the journey is full of joy and success when you balance your energy for health and pursue your dreams. You will find my experiences in line with the best information on wellness published today. I have been researching nutrition, renewing of the mind and putting into practice much of what is promoted by most experts in the field of nutrition and the alternative health community. By encouraging you with this information and by telling you a little bit of my personal experiences, I hope to enrich your journey. My story is unique because I was motivated towards health not away from disease and I have been living this for over 30 years as I raised five children spending less than $100.00 a year on medical expenses.

In cultures past, women learned from their mothers and grandmothers. Today's culture is changing fast. Our mothers were not faced with what we are faced with today. If we do not want the obesity, cardiovascular disease, diabetes and premature aging they experienced, we cannot continue to live the way they lived. We must acknowledge that there were many benefits their culture offered them, but we cannot force ourselves back into that culture. We must live with the culture and community we have today. Let us live well and contribute to each other, growing stronger communities and networks of women for our daughters and granddaughters and for the future of all men and women.

When I first became interested in health and wellness, I read books on health, wellness, personal responsibility and leadership. I found it very interesting that I had gone through my life never thinking about the food or beverages I put into my body, the quality of thoughts I allowed to enter my mind, the opinions I was fed all my life and the impact all of it had on the state of my health and well-being or the power I had over all of it. Like most people my age at that time, it never occurred to me that I was going to grow old someday or that my experiences were under my control based on the choices I made. But eventually we are all faced with the situation of aging and our personal health.

If you get anything out of this one-more book on living well, let it be that *you have the power to control your health and your life with the choices you make.* Without health, we are all stopped at some point in our purpose. Many of the things we call aging are actually health problems that can be avoided. Confusion and frustration are also health problems and they take a large toll on your well-being and appearance. Distress and disease show on your face as pain and tension and discomfort are usually interpreted as aging.

If we move our bodies, keep our skeletal structures in proper alignment; eat foods as close to nature as possible, control our worry and negative stress, get adequate rest, and dream big, we can experience life more abundantly. How to incorporate those disciplines into our day-to-day lives should have been passed down by our parents, but they did not know how because it was not passed down to them. I am evidence that wellness can be a lifestyle. Biological aging occurs but the amount of toxins you carry through life present themselves as disease and old age. Toxins come from foods, environment and emotional stress and need a way out of the body or they promote aging and destroy health.

After reading this book, I hope you will begin to see that there is a comfortable and rewarding way to care for yourself and your health. Ultimately, if adults don't care for themselves, they cannot care for their families or their communities. If we let advertising and convenience control our choices, we will be acquainted with illness. But we don't have to be sick. We can have life and have it more abundantly. You can make the difference with your choices today.

I was a typical soccer mom for over twenty years, while raising my five children. During those years I finished a college degree in counseling and became a Nutritional counselor while I finished a Doctor of Nathropathy degree. I taught wellness and natural cooking classes through my Culinary School, Avenues to Wellness. When the youngest of my five children was nine years old, I joined the family- owned and woman-run business of B&P Company, makers of *FROWNIES* Beauty and Personal Wellness system called Hollywood's Best Kept Beauty Secret, as CEO. Together my husband and I have advanced the company and added a regenerating and renewing skincare line of cutting edge, age-preventing skin care products. Today I have surrounded myself with great people who make the business run so I can continue to pursue opportunities to support women and families. I continue to grow and learn about the depth of the abundant life available to all of us. Through my work with others, I learn and live my journey.

Throughout this book I will present proven information, the renewed thinking you will need in order to change your lifestyle habits, and the new action you can start taking to improve the quality of life for yourself and the members of your family. You will be asked to commit and to put your commitment in writing. This is just for your record. Date your commitment and keep it to look back on and see your progress, years from now.

Do not go where the path may lead, go instead where there is no path and leave a trail.

- Ralph Waldo Emerson

INTRODUCTION

It is my goal to inspire and motivate you to live to be who you were created to be. Life happens in ups and downs. When we are on the up side we feel great, but on the down side we need to learn to control emotions, be present, look for meaning and move back to our desired direction. It was not promised anywhere that there would be no pain in life, but suffering is optional. Learn to see life and its situations as opportunities to press on, experience and understand that this too is part of the journey and has some gift for us. The mountaintop experiences pass and the valleys pass. If you feel your life is stressed and meaningless, you have to renew your mind, just as you will learn to do with food. You can look at your activities and be present while you undertake them and give them meaning.

The infant sees but does not have history to make sense of what he sees. The toddler babbles, but does not know to think about what she is saying. Children love, but do not yet consider the details of relationships. The journey through life allows us to access higher levels of organization and complexity. Each shift in perspective is a new realization. As we mature, we base our decisions on principles, as opposed to feelings. We devise plans and move in the direction of our passions instead of repeating impulsive patterns. Instead of discovering who you are, create who you are.

List the strengths you have, and the issues you can work on. Educate yourself. See your issues as opportunities to grow and learn to overcome the issues. Be grateful for the strengths. I am grateful for you and the new awareness you are entering into. What are you grateful for? List it and express your gratitude to those people and experiences that give your life value. We are in a relationship as you read my work. Go to my website, (www.katwrightnd.com) sign up for the free health tips you will be encouraged weekly. Let's get into how to live a healthy, vibrant life—making choices based on principals that give you personal power over your health and life.

Start today by making a declaration. You can use this one or create your own, but by stating your goal, you begin to move towards accomplishment faster. Print this out and post it where you will see it several times throughout the day.

Declaration:

I am living life responsibly and intentionally! I am moving in the direction of optimum health in body, mind, and spirit. I am enjoying nutrient-dense foods, exercise, and balanced time of rest and meditation. I totally and completely accept myself just as I am.

There is a paradigm shift happening right now in the field of health, wellness, and aging. A new biology will override the past belief system that our physical and emotional health are determined by our genes. This work is a part of that new awareness. It is possible to change what controls your genes and, at this moment advanced medical science and quantum physics are proving just that.

This book is also intended to inspire men and women the world over to discover their purpose and live life at every age, fully and joyfully in pursuit of their purpose. Most women have never considered their personal worth, destiny, or their purpose in life as something to be grasped. Adults serve the ones we love and the culture around us without thinking about ourselves, until we are in crisis. And the older we are, the more likely we are to hold onto the traditional expectations, like those of the 1960s and '70s who believe health declines with aging. This does not have to be true for you. It is definitely not true for me. I am just as healthy as I was at 30 and healthier than I was at 20 when I was constipated and malnourished.

The opposite of this, healthy and productive aging, means turning on all of our abilities; always evolving and moving forward, taking every opportunity to expand our knowledge and put our new understanding into action. Turning on our potential is vital to living a life of abundant joy. The reality is that improved nutrition and medical understanding of brainpower have added twenty good years to the middle years of life. A full life is dependent on living turned on to our power within. That power begins with our ability to choose and stick to our choices.

I share my story here to make a point about your story. My life and my history are only interesting and unique because I chose to find and follow my path of joy, to live my destiny each day. I know; I am the only one responsible for my life and well-being. Many of my experiences are average, but the choices I have made are my choices, not the choices of my parents or the institutions that surround all of us in the United States. In this nation, too many people live like victims of whatever they let control them. Too much entitlement is blocking many men and women from reaching their full potential.

The greatest gift given to me on this journey called life is the gift of vision. I can see what my options are, I can see what others have chosen in the same situation and I choose a life

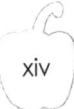

lived fully and intentionally. There have been times when I did not plan or live with purpose. Those times are also part of my story, the part where I was not one with myself and I was very unhappy.

My journey continues as I study and refine my understanding of wellness and premature degeneration of the body and mind, commonly referred to as aging. I am a Naturopath, Certified Nutritional Consultant, Certified Natural Health Professional, Certified biofeedback technician and studying quantum physics. I started this journey over thirty years ago. With every new discovery, I shared with others what I was learning. I kept on learning, and with this work I am now ready to give you the support you need to change your life. If you are choosing to make changes in your lifestyle affecting your diet and well-being, then we are journeying together. I know when you are willing to give yourself the best; you will be ready to give others the best as well. Go ahead. Life is calling. If you choose, agree with this for yourself today.

I am joyfully living a life of abundance today.

Sign and date:

Today your life is changing, if you chose. The change is up to you and your choices. My goal is to teach you the most valuable principles I have learned in the area of personal responsibility for physical, mental and spiritual health. These are the principles I feel are responsible for my success as a woman over fifty, a wife and mother of five, teacher, coach, business owner and athlete. I was first turned on to taking personal responsibility for my life through the area of nutrition. My choices have led me to wellness, joy, abundance and health. My passion for over thirty years has been to be truly healthy by making quality, balanced food and life choices and then passing the opportunity for health on to others, whom I have had the privilege of knowing and teaching. For over thirty years, I have studied and read everything I could get my hands on, applied many of the theories to my life and seen great benefits as a result. Each new understanding of the body and its needs has helped me evolve my diet to meet my needs and the needs of my family. To this day, I consult with professionals in the microbiology and health-care research fields to help understand what it takes to be healthy emotionally, physically and spiritually. I am still evolving and seeking the most appropriate life for me and my clients.

The medical industry understanding of wellness and health is evolving daily. New and more effective methods of healing disease and creating wellness are finding their way into allopathic or traditional medicine in the United States. One thing everyone still agrees on is that an ounce of prevention is worth a pound of cure. I believe we, as a country, could reduce the rate of health problems from diabetes, to cancer and heart disease if only more of us took responsibility for our own health via the food and lifestyle choices we make. Medical experiences and modalities needed for healing cases of degenerative diseases like cancers and heart disease could be improved if the individual was instructed to followed wellness lifestyle principles along with the treatments prescribed by the primary care physician. The problem is the allopathic medical model does not know what those wellness principals are and the naturopathic community is not greeted openly by the allopathic community. In the area of healing arts I find it appalling that so much competition exists. We all need to work together, including the patient. Through personal experience, I know that anything is possible if we will use our God-given gifts and develop belief systems to benefit our lives.

It is my goal to create a conversation in which you will be inspired and motivated to choose wisely. If you will examine your restricting or limiting beliefs and choose life instead, you will be turned on to the power of a life lived fully—the power of your life. The choice to eat to live (not live to eat) and to enjoy health is the best choice you can make at any age. I have heard it said that we spend our life creating wealth and then spend our retirement using our wealth to regain our health. I am intending through this work that you do not live that way. The goal of this book is to teach you how to incorporate intentional daily choices. I am at my best when I live a relaxed, health-focused, intentional life every day. The combination of rest, fresh food, physical and spiritual exercise and productive work that I enjoy, is what I call a health-focused lifestyle.

A good example of this is visiting a spa. We go to spas to receive rest and instruction on healthy living, along with bodywork, massage and facials. However, use the spa as an extension of the daily life you live. Do not make your trip to the spa the exception. The work of this book is to teach you that you have choices. You can choose to create a calm and peaceful environment in and outside of your body, to enjoy the benefit of good health or you can choose to be in confusion and eventually illness, but you do choose. And it is not the good health that brings me joy; it is the pursuit of it and the daily choices that allow me to be me.

Your choices will let you be you or will bring you disappointment and confusion. The purpose of this book is to encourage and educate you to take care of yourself, to take an active role in your health and your life. I am offering you the gift of knowledge, about empowering you to pursue your healthiest and happiest life. Each chapter will attempt to renew old thinking patterns via an action to be taken. You will make choices as you read and establish goals and plans. You will also learn how to handle any issue that presents itself in your life. Remember, the pursuit is the journey and the journey is all you have, but it is your journey. Stay present, be grateful and make wise choices. What will you commit to? Start getting used to writing it in the book and make notes here. My first commitment:

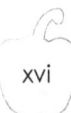

MY STORY

This story is one that belongs to all of us. It is about a child born into a family who lives in a world with systems that control and manage the family. The child does not know about the systems and yet has a purpose to discover from birth. The family is there to assist the child through the young years, to interpret life, to protect and provide for the needs of the child until a time when the child can go out on his or her own and pursue the journey with passion and purpose. The child is potential and energy waiting to discover and contribute. The child gives purpose to the family and brings joy. The parents may not realize the control of the world systems and institutions and forget it is their purpose to prepare the child for the journey. Instead of the parents, circumstances and institutions may begin to shape the child. This is important because throughout this book, I hope you will realize that *not choosing* is a choice. Following the way everyone else does things is living life turned off to your responsibilities to yourself.

I started in a middle-income Catholic family as the oldest child of four. We lived in Dayton, Ohio and we had a pretty simple life and a moral upbringing. Do good, obey your parents, go to school, spend time with family and the kids in the neighborhood and everything else works itself out. Like most Midwestern, middle-class people, my parents' goal was for me to live the same good life they had, only a little better.

Things were pretty simple for me until about seventh grade. The boy and girl attraction started. I believe this causes division between girls as well as feelings of inadequacy. I was not raised to understand that there would be plenty of time for the boy of my dreams. Many of our first wounds (and therefore the reasons for many of our decisions—wise and not so wise) start right here. Food choices are a decision we establish unknowingly at this young age. We console ourselves and our children when we feel mistreated or rejected, with food and usually poor quality foods.

In the seventh grade, I moved from the country to a new house and a new school in the city, where I made new friends. They seemed to be popular people. There was a group of seven of us girls and more boys. I didn't know the rules of this little community and I'm sure my mother didn't know them either. Having come from a conservative community, I had no idea what was going on. I had not been exposed to the drugs, sex and alcohol use that went on at that time. I managed to get through the seventh and eighth grades without too much trauma and went on to a vocational high school.

In 1966, vocational schools were a lot stricter than the general public schools. We had a work dress code, which was very conservative and we came from all over the city, which made it harder for me to get together with groups of people, except those I knew from my own neighborhood. My family did not have two cars, so I was usually in my own home or the home of my elementary school friends. My parents were pretty strict and checked up on everything I said, so when my friends were doing something my parents questioned, I usually stayed home. Even so, I tried to lie as often as possible and get my way or the way of the group, because I really had no way of my own. So goes the moral upbringing while in the teen years.

I have had vision and a preventive mind-set for as long as I can remember, but I did not always exercise wisdom in my choices. I remember telling myself I was never going to drink the beer my friends were drinking, but I eventually did. I was never going to use the words they used, but I did. I was never going to lie, but I did. What is it about peer pressure that sets up the very young to break all the rules to get the approval of others? I have since learned that the frontal part of the brain, where consequence is understood, is the last to develop. It does not develop until the early twenties. This is a medical fact.

My family thought it was cute and all in fun when the girls and boys paired up. I now know it was not. I later learned the other girls and boys in the group were paired up and having sex already, which was why I was out of the loop. Some of the girls in the group, as I know so often happens, were even being sexually abused by their older brothers and cousins.

I was taught about God, went to church and learned the stories, but I never knew I could experience a relationship with God. I never knew God's love and gifts available to assist me in the development of my life; I never knew there was a purpose for my life.

Every individual has a designed purpose and a potential to be realized, unique to that person.

I experienced a typical high school life, feeling that I could not measure up in the area of boys and dating. I was pretty enough and I thought I was talented, but I never quite understood why the boys only wanted to be physical and didn't want to keep spending time with me. Once my boyfriends got as far as they could with me physically, they would just quit on me, so I felt that there was a problem with me.

I went from high school to a community college, working and running around at night without any purpose or direction. Just like most young people in the United States, I wanted to express my independence and make life serve me. I worked in a doctor's office where lots of the doctor's single friends came in with their stories of using women—many of them married men having relationships outside of marriage, just because they could. There were always women available to have sexual relationships with, because there were so many of us who felt that we didn't matter or that there was no one to really care about us anyway, so we took what affection we could get.

This was the early seventies. I saw the manipulation and abuse of women. It was their life, the only life they knew. It was all they had. What I am describing is the typical world situation today and then. I know this can be different. I know the power of God is always involved in every woman's life. God's presence is all around giving opportunity to turn and choose another path, opening doors to better ways and trying to demonstrate love. Without knowledge we cannot see to doors or options available all around.

Parts of the journey were painful for me, as it is for many. I made decisions based on the abuse in our culture inflicted upon women. I decided with the support of the women's liberation movement, not to be used by men. I decided to get as much as I could from my life, never giving up my control. I told myself I would be in control.

Unfortunately, even though I had decided not to let anyone abuse me along my journey, I abused myself with my lifestyle of uncontrolled food, drink and unreasonable hours of activity. I ate whatever I wanted and that was a lot of fast food, ice cream, sodas, alcohol and junk food.

As a result of a fast lifestyle of school, two jobs and partying, I had a very serious automobile accident. I was always tired, always overworking, always undernourished and often had too much alcohol and caffeine in my system. I was out late working and then drinking after a long day of school and work. I went left of center and caused a head-on collision. My vehicle was small and the car I hit was large. No one in the other vehicle was seriously injured, but I was in a different situation. I broke my arm, ankle, upper and lower jaws and I fractured my skull and suffered internal bleeding. My teeth were wired shut. I was in a leg cast and could not put pressure on my leg for over eight weeks.

At age twenty-three, I moved back into my parents' home and they cared for me until I recovered several months later. Now, once again because of my irresponsible action, they had sacrificed for me and showed me the unconditional love and selfless giving they had provided me as a young child.

The care given by my parents impressed upon me the love and commitment they had for me, something I needed but did not know I needed. The time in their home broke my addiction to tobacco and alcohol. I did try to go back to the alcohol, but it never took hold of me again as it had in the past.

Someone brought me a natural liquid vitamin and we had a conversation about the natural supplements that go along with the natural product line. This is the event that changed the direction of my life. I started my adult life over. At this point, I chose to change directions. I was created for greater things than the silly activities I had been engaging in. Life wasn't finished with me yet. This accident was certainly used for my good.

This accident that almost took my life put me on a new path. I started to read books and attend seminars on nutrition and wellness. Wellness was something I had never considered, let alone thought I would lose. I truly never considered what it was, to not be well. Even so, I was not fully experiencing true health even at the time. When you are neither well nor sick, it is difficult to understand how different real wellness is. I made many changes that kept evolving, and even to this day, I continue to adjust my choices to fit my needs.

The first change I made was to start taking natural supplements. The products I had taken just after my accident, when I couldn't chew food, helped bring a new awareness to my life. The food I had been consuming was nutrient deficient, as is most of the Standard American Diet (SAD), so the addition of nutrients created a noticeable change. Then I eliminated white food like bread, potatoes, process foods and sugar in all forms from my diet. Next to go from my daily fare was red meat.

Before my accident, I was constipated and suffered from headaches, stiffness, backaches and tight muscles that twitched and caused frequent pain. As many of my family members suffered from some type of colon disease, I had figured that digestive problems would be part of my inheritance. But once I changed my diet even slightly, eliminating processed foods, sugars and red meats, these symptoms disappeared immediately. The renewing of my mind and the new information I exposed myself to helped change my belief system. I believed it was possible to obtain optimum health with the right foods, exercise and attitudes.

I consumed vegetables and fruit along with whole grains until eventually, all I ate was organic raw milk products like yogurt and natural cheeses, whole grain bread and brown rice casseroles, vegetables and fruit and lots of it. I felt better, lost some weight, and thought I was doing pretty well. I studied cookbooks and continued to evolve my diet and understanding of herbs, supplements, homeopathy and foods for treating minor illness. But this diet and my understanding still left a lot of room for improvement.

When I met and married my husband, I had come to realize all men were not the same and some could be trusted. We did not understand our relationship to God, but we did have spiritual principles of love and respect that had been taught to us. We came from Catholic backgrounds and knew the ways of good people. Even so, both of us had strayed to the ways of our peers and our culture, so that our own ways were a mix of the world, our family's lessons, the institution of the Catholic Church and whatever we wanted to believe. This worked out pretty well because I believed my husband was the type of guy who tried to care for other people. As for me, even when he fell short, I looked upon his intentions. He saw me as ambitious and believed I wanted to pursue the same path he did—family, children and building a home, which he and I both saw growing up. Even though there were some serious differences in our homes and families, basic family values and the Judeo-Christian work ethic prevailed.

So we married and began to build our lives. Life was good. My first pregnancy was beautiful and the birth of my son was an extension of the joy of pregnancy and marriage. Norman grew to be a healthy boy, despite our battling with the family about the issue of no meat in his diet. We believed we were taking care of ourselves in a way that was near perfect. The birth was fast and Norm was a healthy boy. The only issue to take note of was the amount of calcium deposits on the placenta (afterbirth). At the time, no one knew why this would happen but, later I learned it was an over consumption of milk products on my part. The other issue I learned about with my first young child that is worth making note of, was his constant cough, like a tickle in the back of his throat. It started about one-and-a-half years old. I tried herbs, homeopathy and essential oils, but they did not change anything. It did not seem to bother him, but I knew it was not totally healthy. It was not until I learned about the problems with the dairy products he was consuming, that I was able to eliminate the cough. Over all, Norm did very well on a whole foods lacto (with milk) vegetarian diet. The elimination of the dairy, mostly yogurt made from whole raw milk, was the best thing we ever did for his wellbeing. I will talk more about the problems caused by dairy products in a later chapter.

I became pregnant with my second child and was thrilled. I had begun to study and teach childbirth classes and created a prenatal fitness and yoga program for Good Samaritan Hospital in Dayton, Ohio. In 1982, wellness was a new concept. My fitness program was based on a form of yoga stretches along with a supportive conversation about diet, based on the four food groups, emphasizing milk, whole grains, fruits and vegetables. During my second pregnancy, I followed the plan I taught. Most of the work I studied about pregnancy and diet at the time, instructed women to consume a minimum of seventy to one-hundred grams of protein, much from dairy products. Most women did not follow the diet well, so few really ate that much protein, except me. I was the teacher and I followed the plan. I used raw milk and yogurt to meet my protein needs, along with a dairy-based powdered protein supplement I added to shakes. Before you start to think this sounds like a good plan, let me tell you the problems it caused and the action I needed to take.

Immediately after my daughter Helen was born, she developed skin rashes. At this time, I had come to understand that symptoms were telling me something was wrong and were not to be immediately suppressed with drugs called *medication*. In my daughter's case, I understood that since the skin is the largest organ of elimination, her body was uncomfortable with something she was consuming. We usually call this an allergy.

She was exclusively breast-fed; therefore her food was made up of what I was eating. I adjusted my diet to remove common allergens like strawberries, corn, soy and wheat products. I had already eliminated caffeine and sugary soft drinks that could have caused her problems. I used only cotton clothing and bedding and washed her things in all-natural, non-allergenic detergent.

Finally, I went to my holistic chiropractor and made sure my digestion and body were in balance, producing great health. He examined Helen and all things seemed well, although she still had a body rash. My therapeutic massage therapist at the time had heard a nutritionist speak in Columbus, Ohio, one-and-a-half hours from my home. He was from Florida and was only in the area for one week. My husband and I, with our two young children, drove to talk to him about our daughter's skin problem. He looked at my diet and told me my digestion could not be healthy because of the volume of milk and bread (even though it was freshly ground whole wheat and raw milk) and too much fruit in proportion to the amount of vegetables and whole grains. He said that if I stopped eating all milk and flour-related products for six months, I would be a totally different person and my daughter's rashes would go away. This turned out to be truer than I could have imagined.

Helen's rashes went away the first week of this dietary change! Not only that, I had more energy, and my constant lower back pain went away. You see, digestive problems result in lower back and hip pain. Holistic chiropractors know this and work with the digestive issues. Because of the nerve and muscle supply to the digestive tract through the lower areas of the spinal cord, there is a direct association with lower back pain and digestion.

I had physical adjustments, but the ultimate adjustment was in my diet. My constant struggle with digestion was a result of the constipating nature of dairy products and flour products I consumed daily. Even though I ate a good amount of fruit and vegetable-quality foods, dairy products cause digestive imbalances in anyone who experiences back pain or digestive disturbances and this can come even from raw dairy products. We will discuss this more thoroughly in a chapter about dairy.

I continued to study nutrition and wellness, inviting authors of alternative methods of creating health to the Dayton area to speak on healthy choices in lifestyle. While they educated my community of friends and family, I also was able to ask them questions that continued to put me on the path to understanding personal responsibility and becoming all

I was intended to be. As I learned about a new avenue to wellness I tried it on and either accepted or rejected the concepts based on the results.

My next pregnancy brought James into the world. My pregnancy on my new diet, without any dairy products for over two years, was healthy and comfortable, my delivery smooth and my baby large and healthy. I did consume a diet based on whole grains, vegetables, land and sea, beans, nuts, seeds and fermented foods for B-12. I drank lots of water and vegetable juices. Jimi is now six-foot, four-inches tall and has never been ill a day in his life. He lived on a vegetarian diet with no dairy products until he was ten years old. He chose to eat meat while out with a family of a friend. I am not committed to everyone being a vegetarian, although there are many good arguments for a plant based nutrient dense diet. I *am* committed to the understanding that an animal-based diet is not a healthy diet and we, in the United States, have proven that. Look at our health. Countries where animal food is a condiment are much healthier and many degenerative diseases do not exist there. If you do consume animal foods, you should eat only grass-fed, free-range animals without the addition of hormones or antibiotics to their diets. This was my third birth—the easiest pregnancy and the healthiest child.

My next child was Maggie, who was healthy and strong with no symptoms until she started eating table foods. She was a strong-willed little girl with an opinion about food that would not be moved. She ate only whole foods because that was all she was offered, but she rejected many of the foods we offered her, leaving her diet out of balance and creating a mucous condition in her body. She is a smaller girl and the Eustachian tubes in her ears were susceptible to blockage because of their angle in her skull. We tried to adjust her diet to create a balance, but because of her age and personality, she was resistant to consuming what she needed. We tried many natural herbal products, yet none helped. We even gave our little girl antibiotics and still did not meet with success.

After months of not giving up, I found an Oriental herbalist who made a formula that would balance her body's nutrition, even if she did not eat all the varieties we offered her. The herbs were food grade and in a powder, so she could drink them in a tasty beverage like a vegetable stew. We reintroduced the natural bacteria the antibiotics had killed off in the form of supplements and gave her the herbal preparation. For the first time in two years, she was free of ear infections. She stayed on the herbal formula for six months and I wondered if we needed it any longer. But when I stopped the herbs, the ear infections returned. As long as I kept her body balanced, she was free of the ear problem. The herbal formula was based on the Five-energy theory of Chinese medicine and it was quite effective at controlling the problem. I studied the Chinese five-energy theory and started to apply it to our diet. It was an effective addition to our understanding of health and wellness.

I continued to search until I found a solution, because I did not want to break Maggie's spirit, but instead assist her in learning how to use her strengths. Our five children have very different personalities, even though they were raised in the same home. My husband and I were committed to allowing them to become who they were destined to be, within the boundaries of love and good health. Life choices were made for them until they had knowledge and experience to choose for themselves. Maggie remained on the herbal preparation until she was about five years old and any time she started to get sick after that we gave her the herbs. She is twenty-one years old and, today may choose to treat herself with the herbs when she needs a boost. This is what a health-supportive lifestyle is about— **learning who you are, what creates health for you and making wise choices.**

The next birth was Sally. Again, no animal products or dairy products in my diet throughout the pregnancy and again a healthy smooth birth and baby. Sally was named after a beautiful woman I had the privilege of sharing life with during the last three years of her life. The woman my daughter was named after died at not yet twenty-six years old and without children. I was pregnant just two months before she died and told her I would give my last child her name.

I spent many hours with my friend Sally and experienced her fight to heal her body of lymphoma. But when she came to the understanding of balance and its health benefits, she was already very ill and broken physically. The devastation the disease did to her body was too great to be reversed. Sally was able to prolong her life only long enough to spiritually and emotionally heal. She blessed many others as she fought to grow healthy and learned more about life through her disease. Because of Sally's diet and lifestyle changes she added over five years to her life, but eventually, left her physical body behind. Many times disease brings a person to the center of his or her life to heal the emotional issues he or she carries, and such was the case with my friend Sally. Many experts in the healing arts are coming to understand there is an emotional aspect to all disease.

My daughter Sally's birth was attended by all of my other children. My oldest son was ten years old, and he held my leg stable on our family bed in our home and watched his youngest sister crown and be born. On her eighteenth birthday, he called her and gave her a charge to live life with passion and responsibility.

I am blessed to see the circle of life completed in my children. My husband, parents and mother-in-law were at the birth as well. We experienced birth as a celebration. The birth was a healing event and bonding experience for all of us and remembering the event as I put it down on paper continues to bring healing to my life and spirit. My life was enriched and is enriched by the memory of the births of all of my children.

It is my intention at this time to encourage you and to remind myself to make life a celebration, creating events that you can fall back on and receive the joy from again and again. Sally has had a healthy life and started it as a total vegan. During my pregnancy with Sally, I was a total vegan and had been for seven years. Over the last thirty plus years, I studied a natural hygiene diet, a macrobiotic diet and a raw foods diet.

I add occasional fish, only wild caught, and goat cheese (feta) at times as I travel and spend less time in my home, where I can prepare all my foods. Having been a complete vegan and eating many other whole food variations of a vegetarian diet, I must say the primary raw food vegetarian diet is the cleanest and healthiest for me. I have learned that some individuals with very week digestion need different foods to gain strength, but many people have proven that a raw whole food vegetarian diet is the most healing of all.

It is important to study and know where you will obtain all the necessary food to obtain the thousands of photo chemicals, vitamins, minerals, fats and amino acids the body needs. The interesting thing to note is the Standard American Diet (SAD) does *not* provide the many needs of the body and that is why we in America have so many degenerative diseases.

What do you have to lose—the SAD diet or something with healthy foods added? My diet and understanding have provided a physical plan that keeps my children, husband and me free of disease, even free of the minor illnesses most people experience going through life. Our health and lack of disease are not genetic, because both of our families have the same problem as most of America. I have come to understand how difficult it can seem to make the changes I have made with my diet and the diet of my family without a support system. I had a community of friends that also desired to understand and take responsibility for their wellness. For them I am grateful. I encourage you to find or start a group of people who are interested in eating well and promoting good health.

The spiritual aspect of our life is a big part of my story as well. As your physical body experiences health, your mind and spirit also have needs because we cannot isolate one part of ourselves. I believe all the principles of nature have the same effect on us all. We all must take care of the physical, emotional and spiritual parts of ourselves. Even though we don't follow the same path, we are still affected by the same laws. Our bodies were created and put together in a way that there are certain needs the system must have to create health. I am a degreed Naturopath, Certified Nutritional Counselor, Certified Natural Health Professional, quantum biofeedback technician, pain management technician, health coach and wellness educator yet I continue to study nutrition and yoga and incorporate many disciplines into my life. I find discipline a very beneficial part of my day-to-day experiences. Different seasons of life allow different disciplines. When I had young children, the children were my priority and doing what needed to be done for them was a discipline. I find it my passion to learn, practice and share what I learn for the benefit of anyone who wants to learn. I believe it is important how you finish this life and it is my goal to finish strong and help you do the same in your journey.

We may not all agree on everything, but we are all here together, so as we sojourn, let's learn and grow together. There is vitality, a life force that moves through each of us and into action. Because there is only one of you, this expression is unique. I have heard it said, all we are responsible for is keeping our channel open, continuing to experience life and to grow. When you choose to read a book, sing a song, dance a dance, fulfill a position, you are expressing yourself.

My family's story begins with pregnancy. Wanting to be responsible and give my children the best opportunity in life has been, and still is, my primary motivation. There is nothing I have done without considering the impact on my children. There were times over the years that I did choose wrongly for them. When I realized my mistakes, I turned and chose again, wisely.

In my daily prayer and meditation, I ask for wisdom in my choices and the eyes to see the way. I am not responsible for what I do not know, but how I use the information I possess. I studied and applied to my life what would benefit all of my family.

 Today I see my calling in life is to share the knowledge I gained throughout my life with you, the reader, as my new, extended family. I want you to know me and feel my support and the support of our community. You are being born into a new understanding that will create a new life for you. This is why I want you to understand the privilege I feel being a part of your change.

The privilege of transformation through carrying a child in your body should never be underestimated. Five times I have had the privilege of understanding the awesome nature of this and I was supported by a healthy community, including my husband. I knew I was my child's environment. What I thought, ate, watched and the emotions I felt, my baby experienced as well. Having this understanding, I gave myself the right to rest, consume only the best food, engage in proper activity and create a peaceful environment. Pregnancy and birth are a time when a couple can experience their power and influence on the world around them. The opposite is true as well. Pregnancy and birth can be a time when a woman or couple can give all of her power and influence away to systems and others that will control them and set the stage for the rest of their lives. Even during an emergency situation, where medical intervention is needed, birth is a beautiful experience. It is a natural part of a woman's life and the couple's experience.

I believe that the most important times in life are the moment of conception, the time in the womb, the method of coming into the world at birth and the situations surrounding the first three years of life. Research has shown this to all be true as well. I have often considered myself a spiritual midwife and at one time, I thought I was called to be an actual midwife after my children were raised and I had more free time. Interestingly enough, I had a massage one afternoon, and the massage therapist (who did not know me) asked if I had had difficulty with the birth of one of my children. I had not. My births were all quite a blessing and I would live any one of them over today. But she felt a great deal of tension and stress around the abdominal area, and she related it to birth. At the time, this did not measure up.

Later that evening, I was relaxing in a bath and saw myself in a hospital hallway looking into a nursery at several very upset babies. I did not understand this, since my five children were all born at home, attended by a midwife and my family. The events were quiet and relaxed, so the idea of me looking into the nursery was foreign. Then I remembered *being* the child in the nursery. The woman was my mother.

I called my mom to ask about my birth, and it was just as I had seen. In 1954 all babies were in the nursery with one nurse on duty and late at night all the babies were crying and could not be cared for by one nurse. My mother got out of bed and instructed the nurse to give the babies to their mothers. This experience and others like it have convinced me that there is more to understand than we usually experience. This has also caused me to look at my life everyday and choose wisely. It has taught me to pray, meditate and ask for guidance, healing and direction. Healing is happening all the time. We just do not recognize it or take advantage of it.

All the potential in an acorn to become an oak tree only happens if the right environment for the tree is provided. If we provide the right environment for health, we can become whole people with the gift of life to live and life to give. Our biological identities are composed of everything that happens to us, our interpretations of those things and everything we consume, hear, see and agree with. Be careful what you do; every day, you are becoming who you will be.

If you have not had children, reread what I just wrote. The ability to carry and birth a human being is an important gift given to women. Arrange your life to give you what you need at this important time. Search out other women in your community and family that understand this—women who care for other women. We are here, and if you look for us you will find us—midwives and birth assistants or doulas, among others. Read and educate yourself in order to realize the blessing of your life.

If you have chosen to give birth or raise children, take full advantage of the blessing you are being given. Experience the love and joy of teaching and loving a child. If you have been told you will never have children, speak to natural healers and balance your body's hormones and energy systems before you accept that answer.

I want to share with you the story of Jo Ann, a twenty-three-year-old woman who miscarried and then experienced her hormones going so out of balance that she started to go through menopause. Tests were run, and it was determined that she would never get pregnant without fertility drugs, nor would she have a normally-functioning hormonal system without synthetic drugs, starting with birth-control pills. Together, we studied and found what she was missing in her diet and lifestyle. Using a few simple supplemental additions like bee pollen and dong qui, Jo Ann started menstruating normally and got pregnant. She now has a healthy child and a normally functioning body and hormone system. She also understands her power to heal and to choose. The tests told her what was happening in her body, but because the body is always regenerating itself and attempting to create balance, she was able to work with her body. Other women have used bio-identical hormone therapy as a temporary measure to get their systems back to functioning properly. Even at a young age testing and determining what your body is asking for and supplying it while you make the necessary changes is possible and physicians are realizing the more natural methods work better and without the many side effects that come with synthetic hormones made from horse urine.

I turned to bio-identical hormone support as I went through the changes of no longer ovulating and menstruating. Because my diet was so balanced for what I needed I had little trouble moving from one stage of my life to another. I think the energy the body used to orchestrate the menstrual cycle is available for different activities after menstruation which can be used to create anything you are interested in.

That is what I plan for you to understand when you finish this book. You can find answers and health. Do not let someone else tell you how your life is going to turn out or how long it will last. You do have a say in your life—if you accept a diagnosis as the end, it will be. If you use the medical test results to direct your choices and choose health, you will have health.

If you have had children and you feel the loss right now from a controlled pregnancy that left you exhausted and confused, healing is available. Start today seeking help and loving relationships that allow for your growth. Especially during menopause, you will want to heal this pain in your life. After a healthy menopause, women should feel the power that was used to nurture and care for others available for their next stage of life. *Freedom* and *wisdom* are the words you should use to talk about this powerful time of life. Look for women healers who will help you balance your hormones and regain the stability of personal power and healing. All I can tell you in this short passage is that your healing is available and **you** are the only one stopping it. You must choose to be healed and released from the pain of the past. Accept help. Believe in the ability to fully live life at any age. If you choose to commit to emotional healing right now, say in your own words:

Today, I am healed. Today, I am changing my course. Today, I am releasing pain and limitation. And today, I am starting on a journey of joy. Today, my life is changed!

Truly release that pain and limitation; sit back and feel it leave.
Sign and date:

This is the next important affirmation I would like you to make. Say out loud to yourself:

"I deeply and completely accept myself just as I am."

Please write this one out yourself and say it out loud every morning when you get up and go to bed. It is the most important step on your journey to completely and deeply accept yourself and believe that you are always moving in a direction of growth. My spiritual commitment and the gratitude I have for life, as well as the freedom to start over that all of us have been given, has been the most powerful part of the journey. You can start your life today if you will step into what you desire and away from what does not benefit you. You have the power to recreate your life and I am here to help you understand the power of renewing your mind and gaining a new understanding.

I hope you enjoyed and learned from my story, that I was deeply accepting of myself and continued to grow; becoming what was planned for me, fulfilling my destiny. I did not always make the right decision, and I felt the pain of problems, but continued to completely and deeply accept myself, even with the issues of my life. This allowed me to continue in a forward direction, pursuing what was next for me, making each situation and each day my dream day or dream job by being the person I saw as myself. The circumstances eventually show up if you will be who you say you are.

If you have chosen to never have children, then give birth to a project bigger than yourself. Nurture and love yourself and the others with whom you are called to share your journey. We are all called to something bigger than ourselves and there are many callings in each of our lifetimes. We are each chosen to serve a position and to give love and care in that role. Care for your family and friends and see them all as gifts. Relationship is the foundation of life. Find emotionally healthy children to be near and observe the closeness to the Creator they bring. The younger they are, the closer to God they are. When the world and other human beings start to threaten and suppress children, they lose the closeness to God that they came into the world with. As adults we struggle to get back to closeness with our source.

What have you been chosen to do in this lifetime?

To do it, what must you let go of? (*Maybe poor diet choices, maybe limiting beliefs, maybe lies you believe about your ability.*)

What must you take hold of, embrace, to become healthy, or to release yourself?

What is your next step?

As I ask these questions, I encourage you to write what comes to mind immediately. Meditate on the answers. Study the feeling the questions bring about and put the answers in writing, date the entry and continue to develop this thought as we journey through this book together. I have often felt that authors were my best friends. I used their books just as I am suggesting you do with mine. Create a dialogue as we go along. I am sharing my story and hope you will share yours. There are so many ways to connect in this culture—community takes many forms. Let's be in community.

You can sign up for my newsletter at www.frownies.com. You can find me under at www.katwrightnd.com. Check out my website. Sign up for healthy tips and be a part of the healthy body community.

You may choose to spend a week with me after you finish this project. I open my home to three and five-day healthy lifestyle experiences. Remember, disease is a process, so is getting well and so is staying well. Claim your health every day.

If you don't think every day is a good day just try missing one
        – Cavett Robert

CHAPTER 1

ATTITUDE

Your attitude is usually determined by the circumstances of your childhood. Parents, teachers, coaches, siblings and friends all shaped your life before you were able to discern what was true and what was false. Their response to you and your behavior taught you how to perform. You patterned yourself according to the behaviors of your caregivers, whoever they were. That is frightening, but it is the truth. Of course, we were all born with unique personalities of our own, and we use our personalities to determine our responses to our circumstances. Research has proven we have a genetic memory in our cells as well, and even things that affected our parents can affect us genetically, if we let them.

Some of those who were given the responsibility to care for some of you abused that privilege. As children, we have only adults to filter for us and the proper response we learned from them is all we know. A child's mind is like a blank tape waiting to be recorded upon. As they move away from the childhood environment, young adults sometimes begin to see their dysfunctional or maybe functional learned behaviors. As adults with some experience and education, we may make choices based on our adult education and understanding. Unfortunately, under stress, or while running on empty, we may not realize that we often resort to the behaviors of the tape recordings of our childhood. If the childhood-learned behaviors were appropriate, then we are blessed. If they were dysfunctional, we have to learn new habits and unlearn the unhealthy ones. Then we are blessed.

You do not have to be locked into the behaviors of a child. The tape can be erased and rerecorded, but you must be intentional and understand why you do what you do. If the life you are living is less than you want it to be in any area (body, mind, or spirit), examining and changing childhood behaviors or attitudes is a must. If you want results in your life that are different than what you saw in the lives of the people who led and trained you, you will need to take conscious action and make choices daily. This work is to help you make those changes in the area of health.

You are still building your future; who you will be is determined by your choices today. So when you want to change, but feel it is impossible or too late, you are at a critical junction. **Whatever you believe about your circumstance, whether it is true or not, you see it as true and therefore, it has the power of truth.** Belief has the power of truth!

Let us take for example the woman who was sexually abused as a child or even as an adult. Often, this person believes that something she did caused the abuse, or there is something wrong with her. Based on this belief, she has difficulty letting a healthy love into her life. She may want love to work out for her and may be trying to have relationships, but when it comes down to it, if she believes there is something wrong with her, all her relationships will be affected. What people in this and similar situations want is not usually what happens to them. Their beliefs about themselves are too often in the way.

If you don't feel accepted unless you are doing what others do, you will find it difficult to do what you need for yourself. I want to inspire you to take a step in the direction of wellness and personal accomplishment for your own benefit and the benefit of the men, women and children you could influence, if you are willing. Ask yourself if you will change for yourself and for those in your life.

To take charge, you have to know what you want and why. It is important in the journey to participate or, as I sometimes say, play the game of life. Whether in a brief contact or a lasting relationship, being present is necessary for growth and respect. Right now, if you are reading this manual, you are in a relationship with me. I am doing my best to be present, and I am asking you to be present by participating with me through writing journal entries in the spaces provided or writing in the margins of this manual.

By writing these things down, you can start to learn about yourself as you commit to positive change or commit to not changing. Don't worry about spelling or grammar; just get it out on the paper. Will you commit to the necessary change? Will you begin to journal? By journaling or writing out your thoughts as they flow, you discover emotions and feelings you may or may not have been aware of. You may also come back to the journal and see the progress you've made. You may use the space provided, along with additional space in another notebook of your choice but I am suggesting you start journaling today.

As you go through the manual, there will be renewed ways of thinking. I will ask if you agree and, if you do, I will ask you to write out your new understanding and the date that you agree with the new way of looking at the subject. This is to reinforce the new way of understanding or renewing your mind on the subject, allowing you to make choices that go along with your commitments. The renewed thoughts and actions you write are your positive changes. The new thought I am asking you to consider here is journaling. Do you see the value of journaling? I am asking you to write what your level of commitment is right now.

I will be doing this throughout the manual. Putting your commitment in a present tense helps your mind move into the area you are committing to. I will put the statements into am 'I am enjoying' phrase. I am suggesting you state your commitments that way as well.

Renewed thinking: Journaling is a valuable exercise.

Action: I am enjoying keeping a journal in this manual, using the prompts provided.

I am benefiting from journaling outside of this manual as well.

Start these new actions by writing them out in your own words and put a date on it. Answer this question right here and now. You will begin to see change immediately. Remind yourself as you go through your day, what you are committed to and watch it change your life and choices. I heard someone say there no such thing as 90% committed; you are either 100% committed or not committed.

You already know, right now, some of the things you want to change. It may feel as if it really doesn't matter whether you change, but the truth is, *the cumulative effect of small things over a long period of time is hard to reverse*. If right now you could feel the consequences of the future affect on your life, you would change your direction. Think about it this way. When someone is diagnosed with a disease, he often responds in his deepest emotions; I should have changed (fill in the blank) a long time ago or I wish I'd done (fill in the blank).

You have the opportunity to make these changes now, before the consequences are dire. What do you want ten, fifteen, twenty years from now? If you are sixty, it may seem too late to make change matter. Nothing could be further from the truth. You should still have decades of good years of caring for yourself and contributing to others on the planet. On the other hand, if you are twenty, eighty may feel like a long time away, like it has nothing to do with right now. But right now you are determining your future strengths and weaknesses. Just as in matters of money and education, planning your life and health can bring you great satisfaction and reward, while not planning can bring you disaster.

You have probably heard the saying **If you don't know where you are going, it doesn't matter which way you go.** That is true in all things. If you don't know what you want for your life, how can you know the correct action to take?

Write your age below or in your outside-this-book journal, and then write where you will be in five and ten years, if you stay on the current path. This is an important exercise and can be used to lose weight, get healthy or for any other goal you may set.

Age: **Date:**

Five years from now, if I stay on this course I will be:

Physically:

Emotionally:

Spiritually:

Ten years from now, if I stay on this course I will be:

Physically:

Emotionally:

Spiritually:

Next write the changes you know would improve your life.

After you have looked at the needed changes, take this one step further and project where you would like to be if you make those life improving changes.

Five years from now, if I change my current direction I could be:

Physically:

Emotionally:

Spiritually:

Ten years from now, if I change my current direction I could be:

Physically:

Emotionally:

Spiritually:

If you want wisdom, joy, health, prosperity and success, you'd better find out just what leads there and what leads to failure, disease, depression, and despair. **Every one of us ends our life somewhere.** You have the power to choose your direction (the path along the way), with whom you travel, and how fast and far you will go. You are in charge even when you don't feel like it. Your choices today are charting your course. The sooner you choose long-term goals, the sooner you can get started; otherwise you are waiting to be a victim of your circumstances.

Life abundant with health, joy and passion begins with gratitude. Start today, stating what you like and what you are grateful for. If you are having one of those days that seem to push you in the direction of complaint, stop and express gratitude. Your attitude will change and the health of your body will follow.

Stress (emotional or physical) triggers a series of reactions generated by the release of cortisol, which sends your body into survival mode. A surge of cortisol puts you on alert and tells your body to prepare for the emergency, in part by slowing your digestion. Your digestion is the foundation of your health. Gratitude stops the flow of cortisol into your body. Everyone has something to express gratitude over. Go outside and look at the creation. Be grateful for the planet on which we live.

Your body can't tell the difference between real threats and other types of emotional stress, so it responds to both the same way. When you stay stressed for long periods, you learn to live that way. Your body can stay chronically stressed, never returning to normal and, as a result, stockpile food calories as fat. To make matters worse, some people often eat more during stressful times, compounding any weight problem.

Clearly, chronic stress and depression are some of the major root causes of weight gain and poor health. Other contributors are poor nutrition, lack of exercise, environmental toxins, emotional burdens, hormone shifts and inadequate detoxification. Attitude and other stressors interfere with your internal balance, which causes your organ systems to go haywire. This is why speaking positively to correct the stress of attitude should be the first item on your weight-loss or health agenda.

This is about renewing your mind. When negativity tries to take over, you can recognize it and say something out loud that gives you back your power. I like to say, I know what I want and I am enjoying going after it! Sometimes I say, I will not go there…..or, I can do all things through Christ who strengthens me. One very powerful statement may be, **Even though I am feeling negative about** (*put the feeling you do not want, but are having in here*) **I totally and completely accept myself right now and know I am moving in a more powerful direction.** That is what I have used when my mind is really pulling me in a direction I recognize as destructive to my progress. Find a power statement for yourself and write it where you will see it and keep it in the front of your mind.

In addition to the negative self-talk the rush and hurry that causes us to feel stressed takes a huge toll on our health and well-being. When I am in the middle of what I cannot change and I notice the rush and hurry in my body, I turn to positive self-talk and breathing. Sometimes breathing alone can refocus me and eliminate physical stress. There is a taping technique I teach on my web site that goes along with this positive affirmation it is simple and accelerates your healing it is free at: www.katwrightnd.com

Breathing Technique for De-stressing

You have the ability to help yourself feel better. Becoming aware of the push you feel from circumstance is the first step. The next step is positive self-talk or conscious involvement with your circumstances. Some people call it being present, stating, **I am doing fine and I will get through this; I am breathing deep and energizing my senses and awareness.** Your best fuel at this time is the air around you, your environment and the deep breath you take as you breathe in peace and internal calm, then exhale out the stress that is trying to overpower you. This is a little personal exercise of awareness that can be done anywhere, any time. As soon as you notice you are sighing, complaining or just feeling the stress of a pressing schedule, breathe deep and exhale long.

When you return to a private space, to overcome the feeling of despair, suffering with physical pain or loneliness, taking back your power with breath is another great tool. If at all possible, outside is the best to practice breathing techniques. There the air is cleanest and has the best electric charge. Every part of the body is charged and the ion charge of fresh air is what we were created to function within. Use this exercise to regain your focus.

1. Stand tall with your feet on the ground spreading your fingers apart on your thighs, breathing deeply, feeling your feet on the ground strong.
2. Take a deep breath in, open your arms wide overhead and bring them down into a prayer position in front of your chest. Exhale.
3. With another deep breath, open your arms wide and lift them as you look up. Reach toward heaven, release your breath and soak in the knowledge that you are not alone in this universe and that you are worth a blessing.
4. Bring your hands to the middle of your chest in prayer position, again giving thanks and claiming your place of rest and healing.
5. Do this as many times as you need and each time feel the benefit of deep breathing and gratitude.

You can benefit from deep breathing just before you go off to sleep as well, inhaling and exhaling deeply, with intention, feeling your chest rise and fall, breathing in rest and relaxation and exhaling out the day's stress and tension. Be grateful for your healthy body and the better health you are moving toward. Your body has self-healing and adjusting capabilities. In order to access them, you must become aware of the abilities. Focus, be present in the circumstance and take back your power with your focus.

Cultures for thousands of years have used breathing to focus and relax the body as well as produce health.

The health of people is really the foundation upon which all their happiness and all their power as a state depend.
- Benjamin Disraeli

CHAPTER 2

FOOD AND HEALTH

Health, as defined by the World Health Organization, is the state of perfect physical, mental, social and spiritual well-being and not merely an absence of disease or illness. A healthy body is able to function with little effort and it ages gracefully, while maintaining its vitality, activity and awareness.

Though ideal, this picture of health seems out of reach to most people. Today we tend to perform at a level below our true capabilities and accept deteriorating health as a natural part of the aging process. Fatigue, headaches, back pain and indigestion are considered to be a normal part of everyday living and wellness has come to be defined by most people as the absence of illness symptoms. Chronic disease has come to be just as unavoidable as taxes. And yet we do have a choice to make.

Many wise adults today are finding that through a balanced diet of whole foods, a moderate exercise program and a spiritual community, they can maintain the health that gives them the stamina and appearance of someone many years younger than those who choose the Standard American Diet (also known as SAD).

Most of the Standard American Diet comes from the simple carbohydrate sources and has very little food value. Except for the few vitamins and minerals that are added to enhance our processed foods, there is no value in many of our diets.

Studies show the average American downs about one hundred twenty-five pounds of processed sugar every year and an additional fifty pounds of natural sugar from milk and fruit.

About 25 percent of the calories consumed by the average American come from sugar and only 3 percent from fruits and vegetables.

Let's take a look at the different types of carbohydrates. The ideal carbohydrate is a complex carbohydrate derived from starches. Sources are cereal grains, bran, nuts, seeds and vegetables of all kinds. Carbohydrates from fruits are okay, but contain high levels of naturally occurring simple sugars (fructose and glucose.)

The undesirables are the simple carbohydrates (sucrose, fructose, dextrose and lactose), which make up what we know as table sugar and provide the sweetness in candy, cakes, pies, cookies, soft drinks, many cereals and ketchups. Milk and milk products contain lactose (sugar), which accounts for 100 percent of the carbohydrates in milk.

If you are the typical American, you may not eat any complex carbohydrates, but you may consume twice as much refined sugar and simple carbohydrates as you should. The consumption of simple carbohydrates as the major part of your diet is the leading contributor to all degenerative diseases, from dry skin to cancer and heart disease. If you see yourself in this category, make a commitment to improve starting today. The human body is a self-repairing system. That is how we get along as well as we do on the popular diets. It is important to provide the body with good quality nutrition to unleash the healing potential contained within.

Renewed thinking: I can choose to be well, health is an option.

Action: I am successfully choosing a healthy lifestyle.

The Link between Nutrition and Disease

Former U.S. Surgeon General C. Everett Koop shed light on the link between diet and disease prevention. In the first *Surgeon General's Report on Health and Nutrition*, published in 1985, Dr. Koop demonstrated the importance of diet to health and the fact that Americans could experience a tremendous improvement in their health by making some changes in their current dietary practices.

The report indicated that the ten leading causes of illness and death in the United States (coronary heart disease, stroke, atherosclerosis, diabetes and certain types of cancer) can all be linked to diet. What the report also revealed, but was never published because of political lobbies, was the recommendation that animal protein and processed food consumption be reduced and the plant-based foods be added to the diet.

Food is the primary drive for all life, and human life is no exception. The vast majority of our human family spends a great deal of time and effort getting enough food to survive. But just as we must choose to have a good attitude, we must also learn how to make good choices about what we eat. Those of us who have an abundance of food here in the United States must use discriminating knowledge to make our choices. Choice is the key to good health and wellness, the key to keeping a strong and healthy body and appearance.

Because we do have such an abundance to choose from, we have to choose carefully. We are a result of what we eat and digest. It makes a difference in how we feel and how we look.

I will prove the difference to you if you follow the new actions promoted in this book. I will also give you some basic information about the wonders of our bodies and how they function. This is to help you understand why our food choices lead to health or disease.

The percentage of people in the United States suffering from malnutrition is ironic in light of the obesity crisis in this country. Abundance of choice in the supermarket has actually contributed to our poor state of nutrition. In poorer countries, where people have to grow their food or eat fresh, local food, they do not have as many choices, but they do have better health. Our many choices are a result of marketers wanting to gain a portion of your dollar. Your health is often their last consideration.

In the same way, medicine is big business and pharmaceutical companies are even bigger. More government control in the medical industry means less freedom to choose our method of treatment if we do encounter disease. We still have a choice when we choose to prevent disease and create health.

I am grateful to the medical establishment for the many lives they are able to save, but their life-saving efforts would be many times more effective if their patients were on health-supporting diets full of antioxidants, vitamins, minerals and other supplements.

Looking back, the achievements of man over the last fifty years have been very impressive. When we look at what medicine has done, we see great accomplishments. Because of sanitation and antibiotics we have added three decades to the average life expectancy.

The problem—we have not completely addressed preventive medicine because we have believed we could defeat cancer, heart disease and other common degenerative diseases of affluence with drugs and surgery. Consequently, many people spend their final years not enjoying life but running from doctor to doctor trying to preserve what they have left.

For centuries, mankind has been fighting against nature's delicate laws of balance and we are paying a high price for that today. When we ignore the fact that we are part of a balance of nature, we pay the price with ill health, shortened life span, confusion and of course, an unattractive physical appearance. If you take a look at many women and men, you will see that they have lost their physical beauty. Even young men and women (sixteen to twenty-five) have often lost their natural physical beauty. Women are the most beautiful of all creation, the crowning glory. We are created with abundance of health and healing ability, but we need to care for what we are given to realize all of our potential. We do not often stop to think of our opportunity. Instead, we consume and abuse ourselves until we see degeneration and brokenness in the form of disease, obesity or premature aging (which is just another disease).

I have had the privilege of helping many people learn to prepare and eat foods that support health. Being part of supportive communities of women and men who have come together to support each other in making healthy choices has been one of the greatest blessings of my life. Most of the people in the health-supportive communities I have been a part of, have had a diagnosis of some devastating, controlling disease. Many of the women have had breast cancer. Some had surgery; some chose other treatments of many varieties, but all benefited from a change in diet. They went from eating a diet that created an environment in their bodies that allowed the cancer to grow, to eating in ways that did not allow cancer to grow.

Miracles are happening all around us. Many of the women I have worked with have treated autoimmune diseases like Epstein-Barr, Crohn's disease, and other diseases of the digestive system, chronic fatigue, Candida and even Lupus, exclusively with diet and lifestyle changes. A woman, I will call Anita, was concerned about her weight and worked out regularly, but she did not consume a high volume of food and over fifty percent of her diet was chocolate. When she collapsed and went for medical help, she was diagnosed with Lupus. The medication prescribed had the irreversible side effect of blindness. Anita did her homework and found a diet that could offer her the hope of eliminating her Lupus. She found a supportive group of men and women that helped her make the changes she needed to regain her health. Her periodontal problems went away, her Lupus went away and her addiction to chocolate disappeared.

Diet and lifestyle changes do not relieve *symptoms* of a disease quickly like medications can. Often, medications are necessary for relief of life threatening or painful symptoms. The problem is that in today's modern, fast society, if the symptom is gone, we consider the problem gone and this is not so. Our bodies are designed to know when something is not functioning; we have built-in checks and balance systems. Anyone who uses drugs with side effects to cover a symptom that is really a warning from the body will see the condition again, only larger the next time it reveals itself.

Think of it this way. When the oil light comes on in your car, you don't reach under the dashboard and unscrew the light. The light isn't the problem. It's a warning system letting you know there is going to be a bigger problem if you don't check the engine. Let me bring up diabetes here. We have the benefit of insulin to keep diabetics alive. But if a diabetic thinks insulin is the answer to her problems and that she can go about life and diet as she did before the diabetes, her health can be seriously threatened by loss of limbs and blindness. Unfortunately, this is exactly what most Americans do. They find a drug to control the symptoms (temporarily) and never make the dietary changes they should to help support their body's ability to heal itself when nourished properly.

Dietary and lifestyle changes will create change in the environment inside the body while it heals, creating health. The body always attempts to regenerate itself and move in the direction of healing, until it is broken beyond return. Casts or splints do not heal broken bones; they only support the bones while the body heals. Drugs do not heal the disease; they only control the disease until the body can manage on its own. For this to happen, the environment that allowed the disease to develop must be changed and that is where diet comes into play. A malnourished individual cannot heal broken bones or defend against disease. The body needs adequate nutrients from appropriate foods, along with rest and movement, as well as emotional support. Living on drugs without making changes in what caused the disease will only postpone the total and complete degeneration of disease. Changing your habits and food choices will allow the body to heal and reverse the conditions.

It's also true; our emotions affect our body chemistry directly. This is where we find that the spiritual side to health is so important. With trust in God, good nutrition, proper rest, exercise and medical assistance (in that order), we are able to live comfortable lives even after disease. With God, good nutrition, proper rest and exercise, we should be able to live disease and drug free lives in the United States today. Whatever you choose to do with your life is greatly advanced with the benefit of good health. Without good health, you are greatly limited in your influence and power over your own circumstances.

CHAPTER 3

HISTORY OF POOR HEALTH

People perish for lack of knowledge Hosea 4:6

During the time when the Jews were in Babylonian captivity, King Nebuchadnezzar commanded several of the most gifted men, Jews and Babylonians, to be brought to the court and enter government service. The king instructed them to be fed the best meat and wine from his royal table. But Daniel, one of the Jewish men, refused the rich food and instead asked that he and his friends be fed with simple grains and vegetables, quality foods. At the end of ten days, Daniel and his friends were healthier and better nourished than the Babylonians and these children God gave knowledge and understanding also of all visions and dreams You can read the story in the Bible, the book of Daniel 1: 8-17.

I believe the degeneration of the food chain and the addition and promotion of chemically laden and addictive substances in our foods have weakened the masses and reduced us to a stressed-out society that cannot think for itself. I have read accounts of many substances (fluoride being one) that are known to weaken and dull our physical and mental conditions, but that are added to our diets with the intention of making someone lots of money.

Today, the food industry is concerned primarily with profit (money). This is true of all businesses. Why would it not be true of this industry as well? Foods that are commercially processed are done so first to improve their profitability. To persuade us to purchase their product, food companies must be concerned with appearance, so the cost of the packaging is a large percentage of the food costs to us, as well as the cost of advertising.

Then, to keep us purchasing their product, they must consider taste. After all, we don't eat the packaging. So they combine the most addicting ingredients in such a way that we are over stimulated and cannot resist in our flesh. I'm sure you've heard the jingle, "No one can eat just one."

It is only in recent years, and then because of the rampant degenerative disease in our country, that any consideration has been given to the nutritional factors in foods. Are the manufacturers who produce your daily foods concerned with how well they equip you to go about your life? If our food is refined and processed to the point that little is left the way it began, our bodies will not recognize what we call food.

The meat, sugar, milk and chemical companies are in control of the majority of the food industry. They will protect themselves by doing what they can to stop you from hearing the truth about their products. And for the most part, we will receive no help from the medical industry in this area. Physicians are taught about the body and how it works, but much of what they have been taught about nutrition and its ability to produce health is not up-to-date. Doctors are trained to *treat* diseases, not *prevent* them. So you often know more than the doctors about nutrition.

Let us step back to see how things were and how we have gotten where we are today. People used to put wheat, corn, rye and other whole grains into the grinding mill to be ground, giving part of the grain back to the miller to pay him for his work. He made a good living and they received good quality food. It was a fair and honest exchange and best of all it led to good health. This whole grain with a variety of garden vegetables, fruits, a few nuts (usually black walnuts and hazelnuts) and the occasional chicken (when the preacher came to visit) made up a fairly good diet.

Then came the day that a new product began to show up in the grocery stores; white flour. It was a creamy color at first; it still had some minerals and vitamins and if you kept it for a while, bugs and worms would get in it as they did in the whole grain flour. But then, someone found that air properly fed into the flour would separate all the bran, wheat germ and shorts from the protein and starch, leaving it whiter but still bugs got into it. So why not try a chemical, they asked, ostensibly bleach? Advertisements appeared in newspapers extolling the virtues of white flour. What a beautiful flour it was, and it would stay on the shelf for months and not spoil or turn rancid. Even the bugs would not eat it (that should tell you something). Of course, many years later, it was tested on dogs and they had fits, so that particular bleach was banned and another used.

Then came the Great Depression and many people had nothing to eat. A nickel would buy a large loaf of beautiful white bread. It was all some of the kids had to eat (white flour, vinegar, water, and with a little luck, cinnamon).

Years went by and a generation grew up learning to like the soft, white, cake-like stuff and the laws of cause and effect came into the picture. Indispensable B vitamins were not present in sufficient quantities to keep up health. Nerve diseases began to appear: weakness and loss of muscular coordination in the feet and legs; lack of the vitamin thiamin, caused them multiple peripheral neuritis called beriberi.

At the same time, in different parts of the world, men in their great wisdom began to polish rice so it would keep longer. The doctors (in all their wisdom) were convinced that beriberi was caused by infection somewhere in the body. People's appetites seemed to be gone. Surely, they thought, it must be an infection. How wrong they were then and how wrong they are today! There was about one-eighth as much thiamin in white rice and white flour as in the whole grain. No wonder then, that those who were eating beans, lentils and peas seemed to escape this infectious disease.

Next, respiratory diseases began to show up in the tissues of the lungs. Something seemed to be missing that they needed to carry on their work properly. Digestive disturbances began to appear, as well as nervous depression, general weakness and lowering of the tone of the body. As skin diseases appeared, specialists began to appear by the hundreds to reap the harvest of money. More infectious diseases began to appear and microbiologists bloomed from medical schools in droves. Laboratories thrived; microscopes sold by the thousands.

Life was shortened for many and the aging process began a little earlier for those who survived. The B vitamin, riboflavin, was just not in food in enough quantity. Wrinkles began to show up. So cold creams and lotions came on the market. Soon we saw the first super-drugstore. Lipstick and rouge became necessary for faded cheeks and lips.

Meanwhile, in the South, the Great Depression caused many to rely on corn as their diet staple. Large companies discovered that if they took the germ out of the corn, it would keep longer. This is when they proudly coined the term degerminated. The wise man thought no germs must be a good thing. No bugs could survive on it. What about any other species?

Here, a different kind of skin trouble began to show up. It was named pellagra, evidenced by rough and inflamed skin. Symptoms of depression, dermatitis, diarrhea and inflammation of the tongue, lining of the mouth and the whole intestinal tract appeared. Germs were to blame again when a diet of pork fat, de-germinated cornbread, soda biscuits and sugar really caused a nutritional deficiency.

Are you beginning to get the picture here?

The pale-faced white men began to get gray hair prematurely, some as early as twenty-five or thirty years of age. A strange and undiagnosed form of paralysis began to show up and muscles began to waste away. They started calling this *aging*, and we all accepted it as truth.

And dairy was not exempt. Farmers began to take milk and cream to town and bring home a product called oleo. It was snow white; a little capsule of color came with it to make it look like butter when mixed together. The poor people in the cities began to like it and spread it on their white bread. This begat stunted muscular development, dim eyes and lack of mental alertness.

The farmer still had a garden with green leafy vegetables (kale, collards, turnip greens, mustard greens, cabbages, broccoli, parsley, and a variety of dark wild greens like dandelions) and was not affected as much. But eventually, the farmer began to specialize in corn, cattle, wheat or soybeans and the garden was largely forgotten.

The laws of nature began to take effect again. The lack of vitamin A began to take its toll, causing conjunctivitis of the eyes and night blindness. The nervous and endocrine systems were affected. People began to have strange emotional and physical symptoms. The mucous membranes of the intestines lost their tone, so the drugstores sold many cathartics and more powerful laxatives. Stones began to show up in the gallbladder; atrophy of the testes of men and disturbances of the female reproductive organs began to appear. Mothers gave birth to a second generation who had not known whole grain foods and fresh garden produce. And the most serious threat to the human family began to show up as sterility in both the male and female.

Next, genetic experts introduced the hybridization of corn and other foods. Large crops of hybrid corn crops containing about ten percent less protein were raised and this deficient grain was fed to chickens and other animals.

Strange diseases began to mystify the veterinarians.

Women began to fail to have enough milk to feed their babies, so we began almost universal supplementation with cow's milk. Baby bottles were so easy to prepare and sterilize until there was not an enzyme left in the cow's milk. Babies began to develop allergies and problems that did not manifest themselves until they were older.

Next came the transcontinental freight trains and trucks with iced or refrigerated trailers of fruits and vegetables from the warmer parts of the country. A new lease on life emerged for those who had the money to buy nutritious food. Still, the poor stuck with white bread and de-germed cornmeal. The trains and trucks brought a generous supply of meat also; so a poor man had his meat along with his white bread—a perfect combination for disease. A big hamburger or steak of a pound or more, french fries, white bread with a synthetic spread and a cup of coffee or two became a common meal.

Yet we can't stop there. Large piles of bones were left as a byproduct of the meat packinghouses, and the sugar cane and beet sugar companies discovered that they made a wonderful filtering agent to take the vitamins and minerals (impurities, they called them) out of sugar cane and beets.

Then a third generation was born to these malnourished mothers, who had learned to like white bread, sweet doughnuts and coffee for their breakfast. A variety of cola drinks were born from the white sugar, using coal tar for flavoring. At the markets, prepared cereals showed up that were not even equal to the straw used to bed animals. Add pasteurized milk to this so-called cereal, along with a generous spoon of sugar, and voila—breakfast. At noon, lunch is a hamburger and a bottle of pop. At home for dinner, canned soup and grilled cheese on white bread, or maybe a big steak and some overcooked vegetables, with no remaining vitamins and a white-head lettuce salad drowning in a commercial dressing filled with additional chemicals. Of course, they say, the kids never ate the vegetables or salad anyway. Most children eat what is put in front of them when they are first weaned. Give them the fat and sugary foods their parents eat and that is all they want.

It is important to note here just how the Standard Recommended Allowance was created for the nutrients that have a recommended allowance associated with them. The Minimum Daily Allowance is another phrase for the same thing. This is the amount of a certain nutrient that will keep you from getting the disease it is associated with. A good example is vitamin D. When your levels get low enough you manifest rickets. The question is, what other functions of vitamin D deficiency are you also suffering from, but do not show as seriously as rickets? So we are told to take enough vitamin D to prevent rickets, disregarding the two thousand other effects of vitamin D that show as other less debilitating diseases that in the long turn affect many systems of health. Many of the conditions without any explanation may be able to be explained as a vitamin D deficiency. Folic acid is another nutrient that, if in low levels in pregnant women, will result in neural tube defect. Again, what other functions of folic acid are we lacking? We are told to take folic acid when pregnant (even though that may be too late to prevent every problem if a woman is deficient enough when she gets pregnant). The minimum daily requirements are just that, minimum to keep you from manifesting the major diseases that serious deficiency produces. The true levels of needed vitamins and minerals will not be published by the originating bodies, because it makes them look foolish for going so long without considering nutrition as a factor of health. I have read that medical students entering medical school, when surveyed are very interested in nutrition and health, and when the same students are surveyed coming out of medical school, the interest in nutrition has nearly disappeared. Our doctors are generally trained to treat disease, not cure or prevent it. It is your job to prevent disease.

And here we have the degeneration of the health of the human race. The combination of devitalized food, high protein meat and lack of greens brought on heart disease, strokes, kidney failure, constipation, colon cancer and the thousand and one other diseases that have become commonplace among us today.

How have we ever survived? Even with this abuse to our bodies, we still survive, but that is about all we are capable of—survival.

Fortunately, as we have said, the human body is always regenerating itself. What materials in the form of food are you supplying your body with to fuel this regeneration? If the foods I have mentioned are all you know, then you are not regenerating. You are degenerating and hence, subject to degenerative diseases. You must learn what a healthy lifestyle is to enjoy the benefits of following a lifestyle that promotes health.

Let your food be medicine and medicine be your food.
        - Hippocrates
Your life purpose is too important to let disease stop you!
        - Kat Wright ND

CHAPTER 4

ANSWERS

Let your food be medicine and medicine be your food, was said by Hippocrates long ago. Despite the belief that our high consumption of animal proteins creates strength and health, Americans have malnutrition and deficiency diseases. A meat-based, high-fat diet loaded with the sensual pleasures of high sugar and salt content has proven to only produce cancer, heart disease, PMS, infertility and a host of other equally life-disturbing problems. Similarly, despite our high consumption of dairy products promoted as a good source of calcium, we also have calcium-related diseases.

It appears that we are not getting the truth about our own health and nutrition. But what is the truth? How can we know? Due to the financial interests of the controlling meat, dairy and sugar industries we have discussed, studies are manipulated and slanted, or else not published if they say what an industry doesn't want you to hear.

One of the best references to consult on any subject, of course, is the Bible and other ancient books. Although the Bible is not a medical text book, it does have a great deal to tell us about diet and health as well as being one of the original books to give dietary instructions. The food laws given to the Hebrew people had nothing to do with religion and everything to do with cause and effect. Just like teaching your children to brush their teeth is for their benefit, cause and effect you might say, learning what to eat and not eat is for the benefit of the people. It is well-known that, in the Middle East, those cultures that follow dietary laws enjoy better health. Let us look at what this ancient manuscript has to say about food. The Holy Book tells us God has given laws for all His creation. If we follow His laws, we will be all He has intended us to be. The first place God mentions food is in Genesis 1:29. Then God said, "Behold I have

41

given you every herb bearing seed, which is upon the face of all the earth, and every tree, in which is the fruit of a tree yielding seed; to you it shall be for meat." In Ezekiel 4:9, God tells how to make a barley cake with wheat, barley, beans, lentils, millet and spelt. Genesis 25:34 speaks of Jacob giving Esau bread and pottage of lentils to eat. Both II Samuel 17:28 and II Samuel 23:11 speak of grains and beans. From beans and lentils we are supplied with a great deal of protein, complex carbohydrates, vitamins, minerals, fats and fiber. Returning to the example of Daniel and his friends in Daniel 1:12-20. Daniel requests to eat only a pulse made from grain, beans and seeds and proves he and his men to be stronger and more ready to serve than those fed on rich foods from the King's table.

The Bible dictionary defines *herb* as a grass or leafy vegetable. The grasses we can consume are wheat, barley, rice, oats, rye, millet, quinoa, amaranth and varieties of these. Nuts and seeds from grasses are to be our meats. These are all whole foods and can supply the human body with complex carbohydrates, protein, vitamins, minerals, fats and fiber, and the enzymes necessary to digest them. They can be eaten raw or cooked by boiling, pressure-cooking, soaking and sprouting, pressing, pickling, baking and steaming.

The second half of the *herb* definition, leafy vegetables, includes kale, collard greens, mustard greens, broccoli, turnip greens, cabbage, bok choy, savoy, watercress, dandelions and a great variety of other wild and wonderful green foods. These are also all whole foods and supply complex carbohydrates, vitamins, minerals, fats and fiber.

Current nutritional scientists agree with the ancient wisdom of the Bible. The latest research in the United States as well the rest of the world points to a whole-food, vegetable-based diet as the most health-supporting way to eat. Based on my thirty plus years of research in the area of foods and health, and from my personal experiences with myself, my children and many friends, I have concluded that there are no better foods for us from a health standpoint than whole grains, beans, nuts, seeds, vegetables and fruits. Experts in the area of nutrition and science all agree that whole grains, vegetables and legumes are some of the most nutrient-dense foods we can consume. If you are weak or sick and in need of medication, it is reasonable to say you are not in good health. If you are not in good health animal foods cause additional stress that accelerates disease.

However, I do not believe a small percentage of animal protein is a problem for everyone. As a matter of fact, it is easier in our society because of the availability of plant-based whole foods, to balance a complete diet with good quality animal protein. Be sure you look for good quality, because of the big-business aspect of the meat industry; most of the animal flesh is laden with hormones and toxic chemicals escalating the problem of eating meat. It is possible to purchase grass-fed beef but it is not usually served in fast food establishments. Therefore, fast food establishments are best avoided. I would also like to mention that naturopathic physicians working with someone who is trying to recover from a degenerative disease like cancer or heart disease always remove the animal protein from the diet. When the system has gone awry the body can no longer tolerate the stress animal protein puts on it when it is consumed. Natural health professionals in the area of nutrition would agree that a diet of whole, nutrient-dense vegetable quality foods is the ideal.

The Bible and other ancient and holy books describe the consumption of certain animals as unclean. Leviticus 11: 1-47discusses clean and unclean animals, which is a very interesting point since the unclean animals are the ones that many people have allergies to or are very hard to store without large amounts of preservatives. The scavenger pork would be the most commonly consumed animal that carries many forms of parasites and a variety of disease outbreaks have been associated with the consumption of pork. It is necessary to use nitrates and other harmful preservatives to assist in the consumption of pork, making it more unclean from healthy standards. Some sea animals are scavengers and contain many harmful toxins in their flesh (shrimp, clams, oysters, and other shellfish clean the water), and the last thing you want to do is eat from the filter of the lakes and oceans. Once again, the ancients had laws that may benefit to us today.

Renewed thinking: There is truth to follow. I will seek and find it.

Action: I am enjoying learning and understanding what is best for me and my family. **Sign and date:**

The human will is intensity of desire raised to the level of action.
                - John Bradshaw

CHAPTER 5

THE BODIES FIREFIGHTERS

Antioxidants have been shown to fight oxidative damage in the body that leads to inflammation, artery damage, cancer, diabetes, Alzheimer's and many other forms of disease and premature aging.

Free radicals, like most everything else, have two sides. They benefit our bodies, but can be dangerous when out of control. So we must control them. God has built a beautiful system of checks and balances, if we provide the body with the raw materials that were part of the plan in the beginning.

Antioxidants and Free Radicals: What Are They?

The breaking apart of nutrients in foods to create energy and growth, as well as other bodily functions, requires oxygen. Oxygen is the fuel that turns on energy production. Energy keeps our hearts beating, keeps us breathing and keeps us thinking, as well as making all other forms of physical activity possible.

However, the production of energy produces free radicals: unstable molecules that can damage cells and lead to cancer, heart disease, stroke, Alzheimer's and every other disease condition associated with aging or illness. When we do something as basic as digest our food, it takes energy. In the energy-production process, loose oxygen molecules are released. These are free radicals. Antioxidants are the body's free-radical police. There are hundreds of naturally occurring antioxidants in the body, while others must be obtained from food.

There are five key antioxidants that the system needs, and they work together. Vitamin C, Vitamin E, CoQ10, alpha lipoic acid, and l-glutathione are special antioxidants that regenerate each other. Vitamin E and CoQ10 protect the fatty portion of the cell on the outside cell wall, while vitamin C and l-glutathione protect the watery substance inside the cell. Alpha lipoic acid is the most beneficial and versatile, as it can do both jobs.

When an antioxidant finds a free radical, it engulfs it and the free radical becomes part of the antioxidant, creating a new free radical only weaker than the first. So what have we benefitted? This new free radical is not destructive and there is a system to turn it back into an antioxidant. Scientists say this happens over ten thousand times a day to each of the trillions of cells we have in our bodies.

Our responsibility is twofold. First, we must limit activities, environments and foods that cause excessive free radical production. UV rays produce free radicals. Fast food consumption produces excessive free radicals, along with any consumption of processed nutrient-devoid foods. Pollution produces free radicals. Other culprits are immunizations, mercury in dental fillings, lead, MSG and fluoride: all cause excessive free-radical production that translates to destruction and disease.

Second, we must give our bodies quality foods as raw materials to make antioxidants to fight this process. Eating whole, fresh, well-prepared foods provide the antioxidants we need to keep us healthy.

Vitamin C is easily obtainable in fresh fruits and dark green vegetables, which are actually far higher in vitamin C than fruit. Vitamin E is a little more difficult to obtain if you do not eat a large amount of nuts, seeds, and dark green vegetables, so it can be supplemented to obtain the desired 200 milligrams a day. CoQ10, alpha lipoic acid and l-glutathione are made in the body; but as we age, we seem to make less, so these are safe to supplement as well. When supplementing, avoid supplements with fillers like magnesium stearate as the additional ingredient. These are flow agents and fillers that cause a bio-film to develop on the inside of the digestive tract, interfering with the absorption of the vitamin and food after only two weeks of using supplements containing these added ingredients.

Keep in mind that, as we age and overstress our lives, supplementation may be a choice we make to ensure specific nutrients, but it can never substitute for fresh, whole food. However, because of nutrient depletion in soil, it may be becoming more and more necessary to supplement. Many researchers recommend taking supplements in the morning and evening.

Vitamin E mixed tocotrinols and tocopherols: 100 mg morning and evening

Alpha lipoic acid: 50 mg morning and evening

CoQ10: 30 mg morning only

Vitamin C: 250 mg only if you do not eat fruits and vegetables

In addition to the above, I supplement with calcium and magnesium in a one-to-one ratio. Never take more calcium than magnesium, because to absorb calcium, we must have magnesium. Magnesium is depleted during stress and we use it in many of the detoxifying pathways of the body.

Green food supplements are nothing more than powered vegetables and are very easy to digest. There are a variety of brands, so you can find one you like that contains ingredients like powdered juice from organic young barley, alfalfa juice, carrot juice, celery juice, dried spinach, cilantro juice, broccoli juice, sprout juice, dried green pepper, cucumber juice, dried kale, red beet juice, shitake extract, ginger root extract, garlic and aloe vera. Because of genetically modified foods always choose organic. Even alfalfa is becoming poison.

Any green food supplement is great if it contains fresh-water algae, spirulina and other sea vegetation because most people do not consume sea vegetables on a regular basis, although they are a healthy addition to our diets. The benefit of sea vegetables is the micronutrients and antioxidants in a usable form.

Length and quality of life are benefits of antioxidant consumption. Eating fruits like berries and vegetables like spinach, avocado, sweet potato, broccoli, broccolini, sprouts and carrots will boost your levels of antioxidants. Supplements containing vitamin A, C, E, lipoic acid, selenium and CoQ10 may also be beneficial, but never take vitamin A alone, especially if you smoke or drink much alcohol, because research has shown that supplementation of vitamin A alone is not enough and may even be harmful.

Antioxidants work together, which is why eating whole foods that already have an inherent balance of nutrients, is so important. An easy way to boost antioxidant consumption is to add fresh berries and seeds or nuts to your breakfast, as well as consuming them as midday snacks. A fresh salad and a side dish of lightly cooked vegetables will also add antioxidants to a daily diet. Here is a list of great foods you can add to provide antioxidants as a first step:

❖ Berries of all types are antioxidants and anti-inflammatory heroes. They help make your memory sharp and blueberries help the neurons in the brain communicate with each other. (Great food for students).

❖ Pomegranates contain antioxidants, potassium, fiber, Vitamin C and niacin, all of which contribute to increased energy and good health, and have been shown to reduce plaque build-up in the arteries.

❖ Broccoli has almost twice as much protein as a steak, 11-plus grams per 100 calories compared to 5.4 grams from 100 calories in a steak. Broccoli is one of nature's most powerful anti-cancer foods, destroying any carcinogenic compounds that you have ingested and creating enzymes that eat up any residual cancer causers. It also contains indole-3-carbinol, which helps your body metabolize estrogen, helping to ward off breast cancer.

❖ Cinnamon helps relieve bloating and stabilizes blood sugar. A cinnamon stick in your tea may ward off diabetes and help promote efficient insulin uptake. Cinnamon helps with pain and stiffness in muscles and joints.

❖ Nuts like almonds are great for the heart. Brazil nuts are good for the colon, prostate and rectal areas. Hazelnuts help with high cholesterol and benign prostatic hyperplasia. Cashews are high in minerals; promote prostate health and lower cholesterol. Walnuts can improve your mood, aid in brain function and reproduction. All nuts contain healthy fats and antioxidants necessary for good health in all areas of the body.

❖ Bananas are high in minerals and a great food to ward off an upset stomach.

- ❖ Tomatoes are rich in Vitamins C, B and lycopene, while jam packed with photo nutrients and antioxidants.

- ❖ Parsley is a powerhouse of nutrients and antioxidants that detoxify and tone the digestive system

- ❖ Seeds, flax, hemp, sunflower, sesame, all contain a balance of quality amino acids and fiber, as well as antioxidants that aid in their digestion as they provide great protein source for the body.

Nobody grows old merely by living a number of years. We grow old by deserting our ideals. Years may wrinkle the skin, but to give up enthusiasm wrinkles the soul.

    - Samuel Ullman

Anti-aging is not looking younger it is looking beautiful.

    -Kat Wright ND

CHAPTER 6

AGING GRACEFULLY

This planet on which we live offers an abundance of food, wonderful to the taste and in varying degrees of color, texture, and aroma. We must re-educate our bodies with those foods that are good for us and give up those that are not. To do this, we have to recondition our minds to form a new eating habit. To preserve health and slow the aging process, one-hundred percent of the foods we eat should be in their natural state. This does not mean everything raw for everyone, although the more raw food the better and its best if you eat something raw at every meal. Properly cooked whole foods are beneficial to your health and well being.

When this is the case, we will begin reaping the rewards of good nutrition, slowing the aging process. I am aware we all age at the same rate (365 days is one year for all of us), but the signs associated with aging (loose skin, aching joints, heart and blood pressure problems, degenerative diseases and on and on) are not a necessary part of the aging process. Yet adults in their mid twenties have many of these problems and by their mid thirties or forties, these problems accelerate. In the older population, there is an epidemic of degenerative disease that Americans have come to consider normal, but it is not normal in a well-nourished population.

Abstinence from highly processed food in our modern civilization is an absolute must to walk the road to good health and eliminate signs of premature aging and disease, but start slowly. It is a big accomplishment to eliminate one or two food products at a time. Get used to that change by finding a healthy and beneficial replacement for what you used to eat. Then do the same thing with one or two more products. Even one healthy habit matters.

Renewed thinking: I am able to eat daily without refined foods.

Action: I am choosing to eliminate poor quality foods and add fresh vegetables at every meal.

Sign and date:

Let's take a moment to discuss what food *really* is. Every food we consume in its natural state can be classified into one of four groups: proteins, fats, fibers, and carbohydrates. These are called macronutrients. Within each class, the foods should contain enzymes, vitamins, minerals, phytonutrients (or micronutrients) and water. Man-made or artificial foods are often comprised of unnatural combinations of these foods or synthetic ingredients that can present a variety of problems for our health, affecting the aging process. First, digestion of these basic food groups is distinctly different from one another. When we combine these groups into one concentrated food that fits into none of the categories, difficulty in digestion, absorption and elimination occurs. Second, diets rich in artificial foods present a deficiency in the amount of nutrients consumed. If this unbalanced, processed food is the body's primary nourishment, the risks of unbalanced, unhealthy and premature aging exists, not to mention disease.

Digestion is such a delicate issue that there are even some restrictions for eating combinations of whole, natural foods as well. Dr. Howard Hayes' food combining method, devised in the 1930s, has helped thousands gain better health. Simply stated, animal proteins, fish, meat, milk and eggs can stay in the stomach up to four hours and should be eaten alone. Fruits that digest quickly (in as little as twenty minutes), can cause fermentation and should be eaten alone, twenty minutes before or two hours after other foods. Leafy and root vegetables, nuts, seeds and sprouts should form the base, if not all of the diet, and may be eaten with starch or non-starch vegetables. Apples, bananas and coconut can be eaten with starches like oats, rice or wheat. The important principle is to combine foods that require the same environment for digestion to promote healthy, smooth digestion, as well as more thorough nutrient absorption.

The aging of the cells is the beginning of old age. The cells are aged when they do not have the nutrition they need to function so they just wear out. We also poison our cells with too much sugar and caffeine, over stimulating the insulin production and damaging the cells.

Adding nutrient dense food is the best step you can take to reverse the aging process, then eliminating the poisons in your food. Read on and get your healthy life plan together.

People often say that 'beauty is in the eye of the beholder,' and I say that the most liberating thing about beauty is realizing that you are the beholder. This empowers us to find beauty in places where others have not dared to look, including inside ourselves.

- Salma Hayek

CHAPTER 7

THE FACE TELLS IT ALL

If digestion is weak and slow, skin will take the burden of removing toxins from the body and show signs of aging and toxicity. What does that have to do with your face? The signs of aging we all try to avoid are signs of illness and poor health. Skin is the largest organ of the body. It holds us together, eliminates toxicity and keeps out unwanted foes. Skin also reflects the internal condition of the body.

You must eat well and digest your food to have beautiful skin. Limit alcohol, caffeine and chemical additives (salt, saturated and hydrogenated fats, sugar and by all means smoking), which affect the skin both internally and externally. As a health coach/wellness advisor and owner of a skin care company, (www.frownies.com) I see illness on the faces of many individuals trying to change their appearance with treatments and products that cannot begin to change the problems that cause the appearance issues. It is important to use products with quality ingredients that help stop the oxidative damage caused by UV rays, chemical pollution and dehydration on the surface of the skin, but it is equally important to care for the skin from the inside.

All of the previously mentioned items create free radicals that oxidize and destroy the skin, especially the delicate collagen, cell wall and DNA within the cell. Thus it is important to obtain antioxidants from fresh raw fruits and vegetables, drink plenty of clean water and apply high quality skin protectors that can penetrate the epidermis and support the health of the tissue beneath the surface.

I have been using a whole form Vitamin E in an active aloe and oat-oil base on my face every morning and evening after cleansing to maintain hydration and antioxidant levels needed to protect and promote healthy skin. Having researched these ingredients with several biochemists in the field, I have come to the conclusion that any skin care product must have an active Oxidation Reduction Absorption Potential (ORAP). A high, active antioxidant level will translate to high ORAP. Remember, it must be biologically active.

Water is the other critical nutrient in skin care products. Deep within the skin, it is important to keep cells hydrated. This is a combination of drinking appropriate amounts of water and topically hydrating the skin without occluding it with heavy layers of treatment products. I spent four years in the production of our Immune line of skin care products working with chemists to find just the right nutrients and carriers to protect and provide nourishment to the skin cell. Our Immune line is a dispersion, not an emulsion (the ingredients are dispersed into each other by special low heat and pressure) and penetrates the epidermis to assist the skin with hydration and its important functions of protecting us as well as keeping itself looking good.

Common brand skin care products contain multiple ingredients that are known to cause cancer and neurological disorders. Recent studies found that more than half of all baby soaps contained known cancer causing ingredients. When choosing a skin care line read labels and be aware of the many estrogenic actions of propylene glycol, 4-dioxane, and parabene ingredients, read labels and make better choices. The United Kingdom is banning these ingredients and it won't be long before the United States does the same. Meanwhile, we can keep the negative effects of things like alcohols and petroleum-based ingredients out of our bathrooms and off our skin.

Other beneficial supplements for skin health and appearance are flax seed oil and fish oil supplements, as well as MSM (methyl sulfonyl methane) a sulfur supplement that assists in the building of collagen and keratin, the building blocks of healthy skin, hair, and nails.

Acne is a very obvious sign of a nutritional deficiency. The acne may be caused by a variety of situations, possibly stress. Stress depletes the body of B vitamins and magnesium as well as producing a hormone that affects the health and nutritional needs of the skin. Magnesium must be available with calcium and phosphorus for the body to use it to turn around the health of the cell.

If you consume processed foods that put stress on the body, your skin cannot maintain the integrity needed to produce healthy cells. Eat low saturated fats, low-sugar foods with plenty of water, fresh fruit and vegetables. Supplement with a multiple vitamin and mineral supplement containing zinc and vitamins A and C to reduce acne symptoms.

If you consume a diet low in saturated fats and high in essential fats from seeds such as flax and hemp, drink plenty of water and reduce the dehydrating drinks like sugary soft drinks, caffeine and alcohol, your skin will stay clear and healthy.

Dermatitis can be an allergy, usually from wheat or dairy products. Zinc deficiency is often a problem in these cases as well. Consume foods low in saturated fats and eat essential fats (omega-3 in particular) and very little, if any, dairy products or wheat. Consider a vegan cleansing diet for six weeks, working with a nutritionist or healthcare provider. Supplements like flax, evening primrose oil and borage with vitamin B6, biotin, zinc and magnesium, plus antioxidants, have been shown to help as well.

Over fourteen million Americans have rosacea, and as baby boomers enter the target age to develop the condition (ages thirty to sixty), the number of sufferers will continue to grow. You know it's a widespread condition when major cosmetic companies are marketing products specifically designed to conceal the redness. What we want to do is correct the underlying problems by strengthening the immune system.

The underlying cause of rosacea has remained a mystery within the mainstream medical community; however, theories abound. Recent studies conducted by Dr. Richard Gallo of the University of California, San Diego, and an international team of researchers indicate that the most likely source for developing rosacea is a dysfunction of your immune system. Your immune system generates natural antibiotic proteins to fight disease and help you stay healthy. These proteins go after harmful bacteria and set in motion other protective immune system responses within your body. These defending agents can be stimulated into action by either irritation or infection. Normalizing your insulin levels is one of the best ways to do this. Make certain your intake of foods that will raise insulin (like sugar, bread, pasta, rice, corn and potatoes), are kept low. Regular exercise will also help to normalize your insulin level and overall improve the performance of your immune system.

Emotional stress can seriously compromise your immune system. Stress is also a trigger for rosacea flare-ups if you already suffer from the disorder.

Look at my web site for the free EFT energy tapping technique to help deal with the physical effects of emotional stress. Simply stated, one EFT technique is called zipping up; visualize yourself being able to pull a large sleeping bag up over your body. Start zipping up at the bottom of the bag, pulling it up over your entire body and head and put yourself in the bag where nothing you don't choose can get in.

If you suffer from rosacea, or if you're not interested in becoming a statistic of this chronic and incurable condition as you age, I strongly encourage you to consider prevention. That is what this is all about. Think of it this way: science is proving rosacea is caused by a malfunction of your immune system. Your immune system is your key to freedom from disorders and disease. A strong, well-functioning immune system starts with the nourishment you put into your body and your ability to manage emotional and psychological stress.

Most people don't realize that most of the fats in your skin cell membranes are exclusively omega-6 fats. If you consume processed foods that are loaded with damaged omega-6 fats, they will be incorporated into your cell membrane and predispose that skin cell to an increased risk of diseases like rosacea and skin cancers. You should make certain that you have a good source of omega-6 fat from organic coconut, pumpkin, sesame, or sunflower seeds, or their cold pressed oils.

For cellulite reversal a *strict*, no-saturated-fat diet (which means no meat or dairy), is usually recommended, which tells me that these are the culprits in the case of cellulite. Research shows that toxins in the body make the fat hard and cause the puckering of cellulite. Table salt is a major contributor to cellulite while a good Himalayan sea salt can be helpful in reversing the problem. The pectin found in apples and other fruits and vegetables are good for eliminating these built-up toxins. Infrared saunas can also assist the body in eliminating the toxins held in fat by heating the core of the body and inducing perspiration.

Renewed thinking: I can control the consumption of refined foods, sugar, chemicals and salt intake, as well as unhealthy foods, by consuming fresh, whole foods.

Action: I am experiencing great health as a result of my choosing whole fresh foods.

Sign and date:

Ten Steps to slow the signs of aging

To avoid premature signs of aging, eat only nutrient-dense whole foods. Below is a ten-step general outline to help slow the signs of aging and help maintain your health.

1. Be sure that at least 50 percent of your daily diet is raw, fresh vegetables, served as salads, juices, and other creative, tasty dishes. When temperatures are cooler, 20 percent of the vegetables you eat can be cooked to produce more heat in the body.
2. Eat green vegetables with every meal.
3. Eat small amounts of protein with every meal, preferably vegetarian sources like nuts and seeds or fish and other lean meats if desired.
4. Include healthy oils daily, like fish and fish oils, olive oil, flax and hemp.
5. Include two servings of fresh fruit daily, especially berries.
6. Include two serving of whole grains daily, including rice, quinoa, oats and products made with whole grains.
7. Snack on protein-rich foods like nuts and seeds.
8. Eat only small meals.
9. Eat every three to five hours.
10. Eliminate processed, refined or enriched food items from your diet.

It is important to note here that stress is the primary cause of premature aging and many diseases not related to diet. However, because stress increases cellular activity (which leads to a higher nutrient usage by the body), a diet high in nutrient-dense foods will assist in managing health in a stressed situation of life. Vitamins B and C especially are depleted by stress and supplementation is reported to have a relaxing effect on some people. Supplementing is also important with calcium, magnesium and their supporting minerals that assist in nerve transmission, muscle relaxation, heartbeat, and immune function. Amino acid supplementation can assist in the absorption of protein and keeping energy balanced you are supplementing amino acids when you eat flax and hemp. Some practitioners recommend adrenal glandular tablets to support the adrenal gland, which is critical in producing necessary hormones during times of high stress. Hydrochloric acid and other digestive enzymes can assist during times of stress, if taken with meals.

Stress may seem unavoidable. However, only the circumstances of life are unavoidable. The way we respond to the circumstances is the real stress and that is controllable. Elsom M. Haas, MD, suggests in his book *Staying Healthy with Nutrition,* an anti-stress plan that includes learning to release stress through exercise and relaxation techniques as well as emphasizing the importance of a good night's rest. He also encourages good relationships, having fun and experiencing love and satisfying sex. I have incorporated a morning exercise routine of something like walking, yoga, swimming, or biking to prepare my mind and body for the day ahead. Making time to schedule these activities helps change perceptions and attitudes about the circumstances we all live with.

I do not feel like going out for exercise every day, but doing it anyway always pays off. Starting with twenty minutes three days a week will start to pay off in a better way on the days you get out and move your body with walking. Loosening up the muscles, increasing the blood flow, supplying additional oxygen to the blood and lungs translates to better use of nutrients as well as better hormone production and balance. All of this results in cleaner, clearer skin because deep breathing and moving the body removes the toxins that build up in the skin and increased artery flexibility and youthful blood flow to the skin.

Ultimately, a healthy diet of fresh whole foods with supplemental whole green foods and plant enzymes will support the body's physical needs and keep it looking young and vibrant. Adding stress-reducing techniques, deep breathing, rest, clean water, and moderate exercise is the best formula for aging well inside and outside.

One should eat to live not live to eat.
        - Cicero

CHAPTER 8

YOU ARE WHAT YOU DIGEST

As we touched on previously, digestion is the key to health. In digestion, we absorb all of the nutrients we need to function. How we digest and assimilate our food is critical. If we cannot digest and absorb foods, the body begins to malfunction in other ways as well. Therefore, there are two types of nutrient deficiency: when the body is not given specific nutrients (starvation) and when the body fails to absorb nutrients (poor digestion).

Obviously, the latter is the major cause of nutrient deficiency in America. However, there are several stages through which deficiency develops, not all of which are discernable. Therefore, by the time there is a noticeable problem, nutrient deficiency is usually very serious.

FIVE BASIC LEVELS OF NUTRIENT DEFICIENCY

1. The first level of deficiency begins as nutrient *reserves* in the body are depleted. At this level you do not know you are ill because your body compensates and continues to function well. Blood work would not reveal a problem.
2. In the next level of deficiency, nutrients are depleted from the *body tissues*. Still your body compensates and blood work reveals no problems.
3. The third level of depletion is *detected* in the test of body fluids (blood and urine). You probably feel sick.
4. Finally the body displays *symptoms* indicating a problem (pain, gas, insomnia).
5. The last stage of depletion causes *disease*. (This is usually the first sign there is a serious problem and you go to the doctor.)

Three Critical Factors

1. **Chewing**: without breaking down food in the mouth and mixing it with enzymes produced there, the entire digestive process is compromised.

2. **Temperature**: a critical factor is the body's core temperature of 98.6F and the temperature of the food entering the stomach, which can only veer from that by 5 degrees, either way. Therefore, it is important not to consume ice-cold or hot drinks with a meal. Too hot or too cold destroys the enzymes in the food, necessary for optimal digestion.

3. **Enzymes**: cooking food kills enzymes, (when exposed to temperatures as low as 107F, enzymes are destroyed); if a food reaches 122F, all of the enzymes are eliminated. Irradiation destroys enzymes, and much of the food in the grocery store is irradiated without our knowledge. One way to tell if a food is organic or has been irradiated is by the small sticker placed on fresh foods. If it has a four-digit code number beginning in 4, it is conventionally grown and may be irradiated. Conventionally grown foods contain fewer enzymes, if any, which provide less nutrition and lots of pesticides and artificial fertilizers. Organic foods, on the other hand, contain more enzymes and nutrients, cannot be irradiated and have a five-digit number starting with 9.

Eat raw organic foods at every meal and take digestive enzymes if needed. If you take extra enzymes, they will spill over into the blood and continue to clean up the blood. There are a variety of enzyme supplements that are helpful, and I will cover them in the section on nutrients and indicate where to get them. But for now, let's cover the basics:

- o Protease is found in raw foods high in protein, like sprouted beans.
- o Amylase and alpha-amylase are in raw foods high in carbohydrates, like soaked grains and fruit.

O   Lipase is found in raw foods high in lipids (fats) like avocados and olives.

O   Lactase, maltase, invertase and phytase digest simple sugars from raw dairy products and sprouted grains.

O   Cellulase is found in raw foods high in fiber like celery, carrots, apples, and other fruits and vegetables. This is not made in the body and must be eaten in the diet. A variety of herbs are also high in digestive enzyme supplements.

Supplemental digestive enzymes are more effective from a plant source than animal source, because they work in a broader range of pH within the body and can be used to digest food in the stomach where it is critical for effective digestion.

Many people don't realize that digestion begins in the brain. Thought activates enzymes in the mouth that begin the digestive process. When you think about eating, your brain tells your body to start to produce enzymes to digest the food.

Starches and carbohydrates begin their digestive process in the mouth, where the enzyme amylase breaks down the food into saccharides. About 60 percent of food is digested because of the enzymes in the mouth. What does this mean? We must chew our food. It has been recommended by wellness experts the world over that a mouthful be chewed fifty times. Set that as a goal and work your way up.

The next step in digestion begins in the stomach. A fully stretched stomach holds about 6.5 cups of mass. The lining of the stomach is made up of three directional layers of muscles called rugae that expand and contract to mix food with digestive juices. Starch and carbohydrate digestion that began in the mouth continues in the stomach, but **if digestion does not begin in the mouth it does not fully happen in the stomach.**

Pepsin from the stomach and enzymes from the mouth and food (if the food contains enzymes) break down food in the top of the stomach in an area of pre-digestion. About one hour after this, the food enters the lower two-thirds of the stomach, where the mineral and protein bonds are broken by a process using hydrochloric acid (HCL). This prepares the nutrients to be absorbed in the small intestines. If HCL is not present due to lack of raw materials or HCL production blocking drugs and antacids, protein and mineral bonds will not be broken and therefore, absorption is stopped.

Before entering the duodenum, the first eight to twelve inches of the small intestine, the acidic predigested food, must be alkalized by bile from the liver, which is stored in the gall bladder. The pancreas completes this process by providing enzymes to break apart the chemical bonds in food, minerals to alkalize food and insulin to provide for absorption of food.

It takes food four hours to move from the mouth through the duodenum, especially if the food is fatty. This means the body puts in a good four hours of work to digest the food you eat and if the right nutrients are not in the food, the body has to come up with stored nutrients from somewhere else to produce the energy needed for digestion.

If the proper chemical reactions up to this point have occurred, most nutrient absorption happens in the ileum (the first part of the small intestine), which is about ten feet long. A fungus referred to as yeast or Candida lives here to digest any particles of proteins or carbohydrates that are not broken down enough to be absorbed as nutrition. This keeps undigested food from entering the bloodstream and causing allergies, also known as leaky gut syndrome. If food is predigested as it should be, the need for yeast is minimal. Remaining moisture is absorbed through the walls of the large intestine, which is also a storage chamber for the waste from food, which then enters the colon and exits the body through the anus.

It may surprise you to know that inside the body there are twenty times more bacteria than living cells. The right bacteria are critical to digestion and immune system strength. Foods laden with antibiotics kill off the beneficial bacteria, causing gas and overgrowth of the wrong type of bacteria. These good bacteria, called probiotics, should be replaced every day either in the form of food or supplements.

Probiotics are the foundation of digestive health for infants, children and adults. Lack of beneficial bacteria in the digestive track leads to a suppressed immune system as well as a host of other health issues. This is another area where the medical profession will soon admit a need for supplementation in the form of fermented foods or actual added bacteria.

When antibiotics are prescribed, physicians are starting to suggest adding yogurt, if you can tolerate the dairy product, for its beneficial bacteria. The medical establishment says the data is soft, but while new research continues, even the established professionals say that probiotics are safe.

Food sources of probiotics are sauerkraut, natural pickles from vegetables, miso, tofu, natto, tempeh, shoyu, sourdough bread, wine, yogurt and soy yogurt, cottage cheese and kefir. Because of the antibiotics in cow's milk, if you eat the dairy sources it is best to buy organic.

A supplement should contain lactobacilli, bifidobacteria, lactobacillus, streptococcus, bacillus and fructo-oligosaccharides. These supplements are made by culturing bacteria, then freeze-drying them. When you swallow the capsules, they come in contact with liquid and become active. If you choose to take a supplement, take it between meals to minimize destruction from digestive acids in the stomach.

If any stage of digestion is incomplete, the next stage is compromised as well. Poor digestion causes a huge variety of problems, many of which appear to have nothing to do with the digestive process.

Signs of digestion problems

1. Yeast overgrowth, due to a lack of good bacteria; vaginal yeast infections
2. Gas, bloating, indigestion, heartburn, pain in the intestines
3. Bowel irregularities, constipation, diarrhea or alternating between both (IBS)
4. Food cravings, especially carbohydrates, sweets, chocolate, peanuts or alcohol
5. Mood swings, depression or suicidal tendencies
6. Headaches or migraines
7. Menstrual problems, PMS, endometriosis
8. Respiratory problems, asthma, frequent bronchial congestion
9. Hives or dry, itchy skin

10. Vertigo or balance problems

11. Joint or muscle pain

12. Bad breath

13. Allergies, food or airborne

14. Itching or redness in body creases

15. Acne on face, back or body

16. Adrenal or thyroid failure

17. Hemorrhoids, fissure or rectal bleeding

18. Insomnia and chronic fatigue

19. Feeling cold and shaky

20. Weight imbalances: over or under

21. Poor memory

22. Puffy, dry, burning eyes

23. Urinary tract infections or incontinence

24. Premature aging

25. Chemical sensitivity

26. Blood sugar imbalances

27. Heavy metal toxicity

That list should make you want to be sure to digest your food. To reemphasize, it is important to chew, eat in a relaxed environment and avoid hot or ice cold beverages when you are eating. Because the temperature in the digestive tract is important, the ice or heat will disrupt the correct temperature.

The more processed the food, the bigger the stress it puts on the body for digestion. Whole foods in their fresh state provide digestive enzymes to assist in the assimilation of the foods themselves.

Eating a diet that contains close to 80 percent fresh raw food could be an ideal goal to move towards for warmer climates while, during the colder months in temperate zones, the food can be more cooked and less raw. When December, January and February in Ohio roll around,

I consume close to 50 percent cooked, nutrient-dense foods always having something fresh for the benefit of enzymes.

In warmer months I consume over 80 percent raw foods, but if I am traveling or for some reason my food choices are out of my immediate control and I'm not able to eat that much raw, I can tell the difference in my digestion.

There was a period in my journey where I consumed 80 percent cooked foods. This was still whole, nutrient-dense foods. I needed to eat digestive enzymes in the form of supplements or fermented foods like pickled vegetables and miso soup. The enzymes need to be provided if you are not eating raw foods, because enzymes are destroyed in cooking.

Nothing will benefit human health and increase the chances for survival of life on Earth as much as the evolution to a vegetarian diet.

- Albert Einstein

CHAPTER 9

FANTASTIC FATS

Fats are a key to cellular health! I cannot stress enough the importance of good fat in the diet. Good fat is needed to protect organs of the abdominal cavity, provide warmth, create energy, absorb and transport vitamins, make hormones in the body and keep the body functioning. Fats are responsible for building the structure in the covering of our nerves. They are also a great source of energy. Nine calories of energy per gram of fat can be compared to four calories of energy per gram of both protein and carbohydrates. So you actually get more energy out of fat. Fat slows down the secretion of hydrochloric acid by the stomach, which then slows down the digestive process. If you're dieting, this is an important thing, because you don't want to be hungry soon after you eat. So fat provides a longer feeling of fullness.

Good fats are carriers of fat-soluble vitamins like vitamins A, D, E and K, none of which can be absorbed unless there is fat in the diet. Fats help us keep calcium ready and available for the bones and the teeth. This exemplifies how all the nutrients we consume relate internally to one another. One nutrient is dependent upon another and they all work together. If you're just living on one single food or food category, you cannot maintain health.

The fat conversation can be confusing, so I will try to make it simple here. There are two types of naturally occurring fats—saturated and unsaturated. The difference between the two lies in the type of acid that makes up the fat. Saturated fatty acids are those that are generally solid at room temperature. They usually come from an animal source, coconut oil being an exception. Saturated fats are extremely stable molecules. They are far less subject to damage from oxidation, which causes some fats to go rancid and spoil. The heating of any fat or oil speeds up the process of oxidation or rancidity.

Unsaturated fats make up the molecule of the most common vegetable oils like safflower oil, sunflower oil, corn oil, sesame seed oil and olive oil. An unsaturated fat, unlike a saturated fat, is far more susceptible to getting rancid more quickly. Oxygen atoms can easily attach themselves to the open chemical bonds in unsaturated fats and change the structure of the molecule permanently.

Science has come up with a third man-made group of chemicals called hydrogenated fats. Of the groups of fats mentioned, these are the most harmful to the body. Hydrogenation is a process by which naturally unsaturated oils are changed into saturated oils by forcing hydrogen into the open bonds of the unsaturated oil under extremely high pressure. **Beware of hydrogenated oils**. These are what we call trans-fats. Other names for trans-fats on labels may appear. Partially hydrogenated oils and hydrogenated oils are trans-fats. Partially hydrogenated vegetable shortening and shortening are trans-fats and margarine is a trans-fat. Trans-fats raise your LDL, the bad cholesterol, which adheres to the artery walls, causing blockages. Animal foods all contain some level of trans-fats, but processed, packaged foods are very high in trans fats. Cake, cookies, crackers, baked goods, animal products, breads, popcorn, potato chips, corn chips, salad dressing, even breakfast cereals, contain trans fats. Is it any wonder medical doctor's report finding high levels of fats in the arteries of children, ten to twelve years old? Beware that if the level of trans-fats is below 1 percent, marketers can say no trans fats on product labels. This is why the serving sizes have become so small on the labels (the smaller the serving, the lower percent per serving). Just remember, if you eat more than the two-cracker serving size, you are getting things that may not be listed on the label. The body cannot digest them or use them. They are a completely unnatural substance. This makes a good case for a raw, vegetarian, whole-food diet. Not everyone who says he or she is a vegetarian is healthy. You can be vegetarian and eat very poorly. Nutrient-dense, raw, whole, fresh foods are always a good choice.

There is a lot of controversy over the subject of fats. With an increase in coronary conditions, a lot of focus is being placed on removing all the fat out of the diet. Cholesterol has been singled out as a big problem.

Ultimately, you have to look at both sides. Fat is not the problem. It's the type of fat that is the problem. There are a lot of different types of fatty acids. Three could be considered essential (like amino acids): linoleic, linolenic and arachidonic. These fatty acids are important because they improve the resistance of the body to arterial sclerosis (hardening of the arteries), which is directly related to low arachidonic acid levels in the body.

There are three types of essential fatty acids (good fats) that we must consume to get all of the benefits above. While many of us get an excess of omega-6 fats and not enough Omega-3 fats, both are vitally important to our bodies and both must come from outside food sources, as our bodies do not make them.

Most nutrition experts believe that a health-promoting ratio of Omega-6 to Omega-3 fats is no higher than 4:1. Many believe the optimal ratio is 2:1. The typical American diet, however, delivers almost ten times as much Omega-6 as Omega-3 fatty acids. To improve your Omega-6 to Omega-3 ratio, increase your consumption of foods rich in Omega-3 such as flaxseed oil, walnuts and cold-water fish like wild salmon and decrease your consumption of foods rich in Omega-6 fats such as safflower oil, corn oil, peanut oil, butter and the fats found in meats

OMEGA-3 FATS (LINOLENIC ACID)

> Alpha linolenic acids
> Eicosapentaenoic acid (EPA)
> Docosahexaenoic acid (DHA)

These fats are found in cold-water fish like salmon and sardines, fish oils and many seeds and nuts, including walnuts, flax and hemp along with spirulina a cold water vegetation. Plants that grow in Northern climates, dark green plants and spirulina, as well as chlorella—sea vegetation, are sources of Omega-3 fats.

The body uses Omega-3 fats to produce anti-inflammatory, hormone-like molecules that reduce inflammation (a significant factor in conditions such as asthma, osteoarthritis, rheumatoid arthritis, migraine headaches and osteoporosis).

Alpha linolenic acid, the Omega-3 fat found in flaxseed and walnuts, promotes bone health by helping to prevent excessive bone turnover and reduce bone loss. Researchers think this is most likely because consumption of foods rich in this Omega-3 fat lowers the amount of Omega-6 fats, which are pro-inflammatory.

Omega-3 fats are also known for their blood-thinning effect. Thus they participate in decreasing and preventing high blood pressure. Linolenic acid has the ability to reduce clot formation, which is a risk for coronary and stroke patients. Clot formations can be reduced in a short period of time with the addition of this essential fatty acid to the diet.

This essential fatty acid carries oxygen through the body and counters the negative effect of free radicals, especially in the brain. Production of sex and adrenal hormones are a function of Omega-3 fats, but perhaps most importantly, these essential fats become part of cell wall nerves and membranes. Omega-3 fats are necessary to produce flexible cell membranes, the cell's gatekeepers that allow needed nutrients in, while promoting the elimination of waste. While important for everyone, flexible cell membranes are critical for diabetics, since flexible cell membranes are much more capable to respond to insulin and to absorb glucose than the stiff membranes that result when a diet is high in saturated and/or hydrogenated (trans) fats.

In the colon, Omega-3 fats help protect colon cells from cancer-causing toxins and free radicals, leading to a reduced risk for colon cancer.

OMEGA-6 (LINOLEIC ACID)

Omega-6 fats are more common in the American diet due to the prevalence of sunflower, safflower and corn oil. Sesame oil is another source. Usually referred to as unsaturated or polyunsaturated fat, oil sources of this fat are liquid when refrigerated. Omega-6 in the right balance functions like Omega-3, becoming part of cell wall nerves and helping to manufacture hormones.

However, this fatty acid is very unstable when heated, so it should be the last choice when cooking or heating. And it tends to thicken blood, which may cause high blood pressure or blood clots when out of balance with other good oils.

To get the proper amount of fatty acids, mix flaxseed oil and safflower or sunflower seed oil in a one-to-one ratio. You can add soy sauce and use it as a dressing on bread or salads. Be sure to buy only organic, cold-pressed or cold-processed oils and store them in the refrigerator. Also eat plenty of raw and fresh seeds and nuts, also stored in the refrigerator.

OMEGA-9 (ARACHIDONIC ACID)

Arachidonic acid is responsible for the formation of hormone-like substances called prostaglandins, which support a variety of functions in the body. This is a nonessential fatty acid in that we don't need to eat it; rather, our bodies make it from Omega-3 and Omega-6 (3+6=9). A food source of Omega-9 is animal fat.

Hydrogenated and partially hydrogenated oils are fats that have been altered chemically and remain solid at room temperature (margarine, vegetable shortening and oils in commercial peanut butter). These adulterated fats are in almost all processed and fried foods. While the good fats help build tissue and cell walls, these bad fats actually block this from happening.

To avoid hydrogenated oils, read labels on everything you buy and don't buy products that contain them. In addition to sugar and lack of fiber, every snack food contains hydrogenated oils. Almost every store-bought cake, cookie and candy is full of hydrogenated oils. **Do not eat fried foods.** Most are fried in hydrogenated or partially hydrogenated fats. As the oil is heated above a certain temperature or reheated as done in many restaurants, it breaks down, forming toxic-free radicals and becoming rancid. This means that eating deep-fried food causes not only the same problems as the hydrogenated oils, but also adds free radicals.

Also avoid heating good oils to high temperatures. The oils least damaged by heat are refined avocado, high oleic sunflower, high oleic safflower, sesame, olive, coconut, palm and palm kernel. Cocoa butter and butter are also safe to heat. Add a little water to the pan when heating it just before adding the oil to keep it from getting too hot when stir-frying or sautéing.

The fats least susceptible to the deterioration process are those fats with the fewest open-end molecules. The more in high saturated fat, the more few open bonds can be found in the molecule chain. That makes olive oil and coconut oil the highest quality fats we can consume. Other beneficial fats that we shouldn't be using to cook with but should add to our diets in supplemental fashion are flaxseed, fish and evening primrose. These are highly valuable fats for reducing the clotting formation and reducing the hardening of the artery effect.

Proper digestion of the fats is a very exact process that the body knows how to do very well. Digestion once again is key here, as fats and oils need to be broken down or emulsified, to be absorbed or transported and used by the body. As with all foods, enzymes are responsible for this process. Some fats are already emulsified before we take them in and they can be digested in the stomach through the interaction with stomach gases. Other types of fats move into the stomach without being emulsified, so when the food moves into the small intestines, bile from the liver begins to emulsify fat. Through the addition of the pancreatic lipase or enzymes from the pancreas, the fats split into two basic fatty acids that can be absorbed through the intestinal wall by the bile salts and then they can be used in the blood and lymphatic system.

Bile, which is produced by protein ingestion, plays a very important role in the metabolism of fat. Thus a diet high in concentrated, simple carbohydrates will bring the production of bile to a standstill. *This indicates that rich, fatty desserts, high in both fats and sugars, are difficult for the body to digest and should be avoided.* High fat foods, lots of sugar and refined flour products equal no bile, which equals no digestion.

Any enzyme supplement should therefore include bile acids that will assist in the digestion of these other type of foods. I'm not suggesting the enzyme supplement in order to be able to eat highly processed, hydrogenated-fat types of foods that are detrimental to your health. As with all supplements, enzyme supplements should be used in combination with a good diet to return the body to balance. The goal is still to consume whole, natural, plant-based foods.

CHAPTER 10

SUGAR-BONE HEALTH

Sugar is the most common substance that we consume in the United States. It is the most abused food in the American diet. Sugar is in everything. We call it corn syrup, high fructose corn syrup, sucrose, dextrose, glucose and fructose. Chemically, sugar is a relatively simple compound of carbon, hydrogen and oxygen. The value of sugar in the diet of man is based on calorie content and its ability to provide fuel and energy for the body. But we need to ask what kind of fuel?

Sugar is not the fuel that we were designed to run and live on. Our bodies are built to operate on a certain kind of fuel, just like a car. If you put fuel into your car that is twice the octane it needs, it won't take long for the engine to burn out because of the excessive energy present and the combustion of too hot a fuel. Sugar in its concentrated form can be likened to that overrated fuel. Consume enough of it and your body begins to burn something out.

Sugar in its many hidden forms is present in almost every processed food. Authorities in the field of nutrition have differing opinions on many things, but when it comes to sugar, all agree that we consume far more than our metabolism can handle. We continue to do it day in and day out, year after year. The effects of sugar are directly related to deficiency. The consumption of sugar interferes with the delicate calcium, magnesium and potassium balance necessary for virtually every bodily function from running to sleeping.

Volumes have been written on sugar consumption and human metabolism. Thirty years ago, our parents told us that sugar rots our teeth and today we know that is the least of the problems. No substance that we readily consume is as addictive. We've all heard of diabetes and hypoglycemia, two common and serious disorders linked directly to sugar consumption and metabolism. The medical profession has labeled hypoglycemia as the physiological disorder of our time. In recent years, biochemists have been able to show just how common this condition really is. Hypoglycemia is really the physiological manifestation of a sugar addiction. As glucose is cut off or reduced in normal amounts, the body reacts with panic. The whole reaction is chemical and is hidden inside the body tissue. For this reason, few people are ready to deal with the many side effects. As the war between sugar and insulin continues, the addiction worsens. Common symptoms of hypoglycemia include hunger, dizziness, irritability, nausea, anxiety, tremors and panic attacks.

The list of sugar-abused disorders goes on: acne, tooth decay, obesity, elevated cholesterol levels, gingivitis, cardiovascular disease and a host of mental and emotional disorders. Oriental visual diagnosis reports the effects of sugar on the liver and digestive organs, as it leaves lines on the forehead and between the eyes, both vertical and horizontal. Sugar shows on your face. Fatigue, circles around the eyes, sometimes allergies to other foods and the telltale puffy bags under the corners of the lower eyes are often times allergies that are created by sugar. Alcohol is an especially strong culprit. If you go out one night and have a few drinks, the next morning when you get up, your eyes are puffy.

Sugar is the most consumed and the least understood food in the Standard American Diet (also known as SAD). Most people consume their own weight in sugar in one year. So the average young adult woman who weighs between 125-150 pounds consumes between 125-150 pounds of sugar or more each year! After doing this for five to ten years, that average woman will no longer be average. She will have added at least five to ten pounds per year, a fifty to one-hundred-pound weight gain. If she started in her twenties weighing 125 pounds, she could easily end up in her thirties and early forties at 225 pounds and laden with disease.

Processed foods account for more than 90 percent of the money Americans spend on their meals. About **one-quarter of the calories consumed by the average American is in the form of added sugars,** the majority of which comes from high fructose corn syrup (HFCS) as a category of sugar by itself.

Part of what makes HFCS such a dangerous sweetener is that it is metabolized to fat in your body far more rapidly than any other sugar. According to Dr. Elizabeth Parks, associate professor of clinical nutrition at University of Texas Southwestern Medical Center and lead author of a study on fructose, published in the *Journal of Nutrition,* our study shows for the first time the surprising speed with which humans make body fat from fructose. Once you start the process of fat synthesis from fructose, it's hard to slow it down. The bottom line of this study is that fructose very quickly gets made into fat in your body

This occurs because most fats are formed in the liver. When sugar enters it, the liver decides whether to store it, burn it, or turn it into fat. Fructose, however, bypasses this process and simply turns into fat. Studies published to date on this topic also found that fructose consumption leads to decreased signaling to the central nervous system from the hormones leptin and insulin, which act as key signals in regulating how much we eat, as well as body weight. This suggests that dietary fructose may contribute to increased food intake and weight gain. Decreased insulin and leptin signaling is also a main cause of diabetes and a host of other obesity-related conditions.

What's the bottom line here? **Avoid high fructose corn syrup at all costs.**

Treat it like poison. If you do purchase packaged foods, become an avid label reader and avoid foods that contain corn syrup as a main ingredient.

Take a minute right now to consider what you just read. Do you believe it? If not, do your own research. Much research on the topic of sugar says high fructose corn sweetener is not different than any other sugar, but it is important to note that much of the funding for these studies comes from organizations with a financial interest in high fructose corn sweeteners. You will find two opinions about diet and lifestyle in our culture. One says to eat whatever you want: eat, drink, and be merry, for then you shall surely die. It's true! You will die, sooner and sicker. The other opinion encourages us to enjoy all things in moderation and know what effect they have on our bodies.

Test this for yourself. First abstain from the food in question, in this case sugar, for at least six weeks. You will find out if you can abstain. If not, there is surely an addictive, controlling nature to the substance. If you can abstain, after the six-week fast, eat plenty of the substance and see how it affects your body. You will be the true judge. We are, after all, responsible for our life and health. You can give your responsibility away, but I am suggesting you choose not to do that.

Usually there is an emotional attachment to refined foods. Like alcohol, all refined sugar foods give an emotional reaction and comfort we do not realize until we have tried to give them up. If you do believe you have a problem with refined sugars, stop and think about this. **Are you ready to take control?** Write it down here:

List the reasons why you do or do not believe sugar is a problem food. Your mind should tell you when you are ready to take back your power. Renewing your mind with information and new beliefs is the first step you must take before change is lasting.

Renewed thinking: Right now I acknowledge I can have power over sugar in my life.

Action: I am benefiting abundantly from my choice to limit my consumption of sugar.

Sign and date:

One simple way to reduce your sugar intake is to stay away from the sugar bowl. It is not necessary to add sugar to foods that are already heavily sweetened. Each rounded teaspoon of sugar weighs approximately nine grams. Every time we stop and don't add sugar, we consume nine grams less of it.

Prepared breakfast cereals, as well as sweet desserts, are a large part of highly concentrated sugars. That doesn't mean that you can't enjoy a sweet dessert occasionally, but quantity is the key to the problem. With sugar, more is definitely not better. Soft drinks are another concentrated sugar. Most soft drinks use high fructose corn sugar. Each soft drink contains between five and seven tablespoons of pure sugar. How many do you think most people drink on an average hot day? Sugar adds up quickly. Most soft drinks are sweetened with high fructose corn sweetener (HFCS) as well. There are about forty grams of HFCS per can of soda beverages—more that the American Medical Association's recommended daily maximum for ALL caloric sweeteners. High-fructose diets have been linked to hypertriglyceridemia, nonalcoholic fatty liver disease (insulin resistance leading to diabetes).

There are alternatives to soft drinks and desserts, but non-caloric, artificial sweeteners are not the answer. Since the introduction of artificial sweeteners, Americans have gained weight. These sweeteners have been shown to increase weight when given to animals and are believed to stimulate undesirable brain chemicals that cause oxidative damage to brain cells.

Stevia is a plant with very sweet leaves; an extract from those leaves will sweeten an iced herbal tea or carbonated water. It is so concentrated that only a couple of drops are equal to several teaspoons of sugar with none of the devastating side effects. It actually has benefits. It is said to regulate blood sugar levels and herbalists consider it an antibacterial, antiviral and antifungal agent. I have used stevia in herbal teas for over ten years now. I don't get headaches, but often I have been with someone struggling with a headache or blood sugar drops that cause fatigue or dizziness. When I share my stevia, I have seen it relieve their symptoms every time.

Several brands of decaffeinated green tea extracts sweetened with stevia or flavored with fruit are available. I buy Pure Inventions Green Tea Extracts. You can find them on the resource page of my Web site, www.katwrightnd.com.

There are additional benefits to a drink like this. Besides the reduction of sugar, the phenols in green tea contribute to immune health. Phenols are strong antioxidants that fight free radicals. If you remember, free radicals lead to inflammation and tissue damage.

Renewed thinking: I can control my choice of beverage.

Action: I am enjoying the taste and benefit of stevia-sweetened beverages.

Sign and date:

There are many forms of hidden sugar in foods we might consider to be innocent. Any white carbohydrate is a hidden sugar. Processed foods containing refined flour labeled wheat flour, unbleached wheat flour or any other starchy, processed grain is converted immediately into sugar in the body. So those white breads, bagels, wraps, pretzels, potato chips, pancakes, waffles and donuts are all simple sugars (carbohydrates) contributing to high blood sugar, that leads to low blood sugar, that leads to problems. Diabetics are told not to eat carbohydrates for this reason. The reality is that the body needs carbohydrates, but in their whole form. Processed foods have these valuable nutrients removed.

To keep your glucose (blood sugar) level steady and healthy, reduce the amount of processed foods in your diet until you have eliminated them. I have seen many people reduce the harmful foods and think that is good enough, but over time, processed foods creep back to the levels they were before the changes are ever considered. Make it your goal to reduce them until they are eliminated. Keep in mind that fruit juice is a processed food and high in simple sugars.

Renewed thinking: I can learn which foods have hidden sugars.

Action: I am eliminating hidden sugars and processed foods

Sign and date:

Consuming foods with high levels of magnesium and potassium will help regulate blood sugar levels. Eat good quality whole grains in the morning and eliminate any processed refined grains. Purchase natural health food brands that list all ingredients and are organically grown. Make sure breakfast cereals are without added sugar. Try a combination of soft cooked whole oats, rice and millet, and eat them with added fruit and nuts. By adding ground flax or hemp seeds, you increase the protein and Omega-3 and Omega-6 in your diet and greatly benefit your blood sugar levels. If you feel the need to sweeten the taste, use a small amount of stevia or rice syrup. Remember, stevia is very concentrated—a small amount goes a long way.

Renewed thinking: I can take back control from the sugar industry and make healthy choices in breakfast cereal starting today.

Action: I am making healthy choices at breakfast, lunch, dinner and snacks.

Sign and date:

Remember, sugar is addicting. We usually recognize a candy bar and soft drink addiction or an alcohol addiction, but most people do not realize they are physically addicted to bread, pasta and potatoes. If you have the above listed items more often than once a month, you are affecting your blood sugar levels and your body's health. This is the first place to start changing your life nutritionally.

It's important to acknowledge that advertising and social habits have influenced your eating habits. Everyone you know stops for coffee or bagels in the morning and you want to be like them. But do you want their health? Many people are able to eat that way and not gain weight, so they think they are fine. This is deceptive. No one is fine when the nutrients needed to produce healthy hormone balance and body function are missing. They are like a time bomb waiting to explode.

Renewed thinking: I can take control over convincing advertising. I will not let advertising control my food choices.

Action: I am learning and applying better ways of caring for myself.

Sign and date:

A journey of a thousand miles begins with a single step
- Chinese proverb

CHAPTER 11

GENUINE SALT

Genuine sea salt is composed of minerals from the ocean which have been transformed by microorganisms, algae and plants into organic nutrients. It supplies all 92 vital trace elements harmoniously combined to promote optimum biological functioning and cellular maintenance.

A combination of sodium and chloride, two common and essential substances, in fact, sodium chloride, common table salt, is actually necessary in the human diet. However, as with sugar, the problem with salt lies in the quantity and quality. It is estimated that approximately one-third of a gram of salt is the amount needed by the body each day. This amount can be easily obtained through common foods such as vegetables and fruits. However, today, the average American consumes an average of ten to fifteen grams of salt per day.

Modern packaging and processing has caused us to consume more salt than ever. It is a very inexpensive preservative and, as such, is added to practically every food during processing. So we should reduce our consumption of salt whenever possible. One way to do that is to, once again, reduce consumption of processed foods and instead eat foods closer to their natural state. Interestingly, this is the same action taken to help control the consumption of excess sugar.

Just like sugar, salt causes swelling in the face. It causes you to hold water around the eyes, it causes problems in elimination through the skin, and it causes problems with bacterial growth. It causes all types of problems with appearance. Salt seems to have a detrimental effect on a great many functions of the body. We know that salt retards the digestion and the assimilation of protein, primarily because of the reduction effect it has on the protein enzyme pepsin. So we don't digest protein well when we consume salt, yet how many people salt their chicken and their steak and their eggs?

Another common ill effect from an imbalance of sodium chloride is hypertension. Salt may be the single greatest cause of high blood pressure. This is substantiated by studies that show a direct correlation between salt consumption and the incidents of hypertension in varying ethnic groups. When people who have not consumed a high amount of sodium chloride in the past increase their consumption, these same diseases show up.

Kidney function is drastically hindered through the use of salt. The kidneys eliminate salt from the body, keeping electrolytes balanced. Great stress is placed on the kidneys when they must continually dilute and eliminate an excess of concentrated salt. From an anti-aging standpoint, we age the body when we overwork it. If we burn an engine too hot, we end up burning out the engine sooner than its intended life. The same thing is true with our bodies. If we over-consume salt and overwork the kidneys, it causes the aging process of the skin to accelerate.

One of the most common side effects of overindulgence of salt is swelling, or edema. The kidneys cannot eliminate the volume of salt that we ingest, so the tissue becomes waterlogged, which is the body's defense mechanism against salt-laden cells. Water is flooded into the tissue to dilute the salt concentration. A simple test to find out if your body has an over abundance of salt is to taste your perspiration. If it tastes very salty, you're perspiring in order to eliminate sodium chloride from your system. Salt loss through perspiration does not need to be replaced through direct consumption of more salt. We obtain more than an ample supply of salt through our daily consumption of food. The expiration of salt by sweating is beneficial to the body. It regulates the balance between the elements very rapidly.

There are many ways to reduce salt intake. When salt is added to food, it should be added using unrefined sea salt and cooked into the food. Unrefined sea salt is only 40 percent sodium, and the rest is made of trace elements and minerals beneficial to the body. Salt is necessary for many functions of the body, such as allowing fluids to pass in and out of your cells, carrying nutrients, and helping the cells in your brain and body transfer information as well as regulating blood pressure. You need some salt but only unrefined.

I consume Himalayan sea salt to re-mineralize my body. You can find Himalayan salt on my Web site (www.katwrightnd.com). Food sources of salt are alfalfa, celery, carrots, sea vegetables, beets and raw, green, leafy vegetables. You can also use additional herbs and spices to give food flavor. The taste of salt is habitual, so be careful. Salty foods dilute the taste buds of the mouth to taste anything but salt. All the finer tastes are no longer detected by the taste buds because we habitually use salt. Consequently, we pour on the salt because of the lack of taste. Salt also interferes with protein digestion, but who eats their steaks, chicken or burgers without salt?

Turmeric is an herb that has been traditionally used in India to season foods. Recently it has been discovered that turmeric has an array of antioxidant, anti-cancer, antibiotic, antiviral and other beneficial properties. In India, they call turmeric holy powder because of its broad range of health benefits, including strengthening and improving digestion, purifying the blood, anti-inflammatory properties, anti-cancer properties, arthritis prevention and aiding against Alzheimer's disease. Turmeric is a beneficial seasoning to choose over salt.

There can be signs of a deficiency in good quality salt. Some common deficiency signs include low blood sugar, muscle degeneration, irregular heartbeat, hypertension, depleted potassium, stiff joints, floaters in the eyes, and thin or nonexistent mucous membranes.

Renewed thinking: I can eliminate table salt from my diet.

Action: I am using good quality sea salt on my food.

Sign and date:

With all the evidence thus far against processed foods and against overconsumption of sugar and salt, here are a few recommendations:

Avoid fast food and junk foods: These foods all contain white flour, sugar, salt, hydrogenated oils (trans-fats) and tons of preservatives and additives to enhance the taste. It is questionable whether these foods are food at all. They leave you feeling tired, make you fat and disturb your biochemistry.

Avoid foods you are addicted to. Foods you crave and must have usually have a destructive affect on your body. List the foods you must have:

Renewed thinking: Processed, refined foods are high in poor quality, health-damaging oils, as well as hidden sugars and salt. Processed foods and snack foods are deceptive and deprive me of what I need to be healthy.

Action: I am reading labels and finding whole, healthy foods and snacks to support my body.

Sign and date:

Ask yourself these questions:

Am I ready to stop eating food that damages my health?
Am I ready to add health-supportive foods to my diet?
When will I begin?
Who will hold me accountable?
What will get in my way?
What do I expect to accomplish?
Will I change immediately or gradually?

CHAPTER 12

PROTEIN

Protein comes from a Greek word meaning, "of first importance." All of the structural material of the body is built out of protein and the building blocks of protein itself are called amino acids. Every reaction that takes place in the body's nervous, digestive, muscular, or circulatory system is directly related to and dependent on these amino acids in the body. Children especially require high protein diets to carry out the different building processes that are going on in their bodies. Similarly, a pregnant woman requires a high protein diet in order to carry out the building process of the child that she is carrying.

But even after the body has formed and grown, need for protein is primary. It's the quality and again the quantity, or volume of protein that we need to consider. Living tissue is in a constant state of breaking down and needs to be rebuilt, which means that the building blocks, amino acids, are constantly being exchanged for new amino acid combinations. Blood carries these amino acids where they need to go in the body. If the available source of amino acids runs low, the blood in its delivery role will actually leech protein from the surrounding tissue to deliver it somewhere else. That leaves some tissue in less than an optimal state. So you can see how muscle tissue becomes lacking as we age if the protein has to be taken out of it, and we'll have slack, loose skin that makes us look older.

If sufficient protein is not provided, this process continues. When muscle tissue is not available, organs can actually be damaged by the absence of protein in the diet. A deficiency of quality protein is a serious crisis for a functioning, healthy body and the body cannot persevere under a permanent deficit of protein.

But diets too high in protein can also cause problems. If you consume too much protein, you send your body into a condition called ketosis. The body starts to consume itself, which can again damage organs. Too much protein also causes an acidosis condition in the blood, leading to the leeching of calcium from the bones to alkalinize the acid condition of the blood. So it's important that we don't consume any one food group in excess but that we balance them all.

Proteins are one of the most complex organic compounds in nature. Digestion of a complex molecule is accomplished in several very distinct and important phases. As we've discussed, protein digestion begins in the stomach. Hydrochloric acid and protease enzymes from the pancreas break down the complete molecules of protein into their separate amino acids, so they can be absorbed or assimilated into the body through the intestinal wall. An important note: intact proteins are not supposed to be absorbed into the blood, and if they are, some very serious side effects occur. The lack of digestive enzymes provided by the body and the foods we eat leaves protein undigested as it moves through the digestive process. In the last stage of digestion a micro organism, referred to as yeast, is present to assist in the breakdown of foods in their undigested state. If this is a common problem, yeast becomes an overgrowth and causes many of its own health-related problems. At this stage of digestion, some proteins may move through the gut wall and set the body up for allergies and painful conditions that remain difficult for the medical profession to diagnose. The absorption of a whole protein most commonly creates an allergic reaction. To avoid this problem, it is important to consider the diet and the types of foods consumed. It is also important to proper digestion that we choose nutrient-dense foods that provide the body with the critical nutrients for proper function. Chewing those foods in a relaxed environment is equally valuable to proper digestion. Since digestion is so critical to the proper assimilation of proteins, the digestion function should be a great concern to us.

At about age thirty-five, many people suffer from a reduction in the natural production of hydrochloric acid in their digestive tract. This happens because, when we are younger, we assault the digestive tract with such poor foods that there is no enzyme support left in our body. In light of this, enzyme supplements are often required. Whatever formula you choose should contain, not only the hydrochloric acid and pepsin that you need for protein, but also a broad spectrum of enzyme support so that all types of foods including fats and carbohydrates can be digested.

There are many options for obtaining the amount of protein you need. I will give a complete list at the end of the foods section, but for now, these categories will suffice: beef, poultry, fish, nuts, grains, seeds and beans. Most vegetables and grains also contain small amounts of protein. As a result, we usually get too much protein because of its abundance in the United States. Therefore, our action here is to pay attention and limit the amount of protein to appropriate body weight amounts unless you are pregnant, nursing or a child.

You can obtain enough protein from a whole foods, plant-based diet. In fact, most animals build their muscles from plant proteins. I want to emphasize the importance of balance if you chose to be vegan. I chose to be a vegan for seventeen years and they were the healthiest seventeen years of my life. I gave birth to three of my five children as a vegan. The birth and child were healthy every time. It is important to tell you I spent my time being sure my protein and other nutrients were available to me and my other children.

At this time I do occasionally consume fish when I travel, when I am not able to get quality vegetarian protein. At this time in history, there are so many more great vegetarian restaurants that it has become easier to travel and maintain a healthy vegan diet. One thing I must mention about being vegan, it is usually necessary to take a vitamin B-12 supplement unless you make your own fermented foods on a regular basis.

Fermented foods may be reported to contain B-12, but, B-12 is only found in animal products. The fermentation of soy products contains beneficial bacteria that in some cases have been shown to contain B-12. Because commercially made food products differ from the traditional fermented products in the serialization necessary for sanitation, it is unlikely you will find B-12. Bee pollen may be a natural source of B-12 and other health-supportive properties as well. Bee pollen has more amino acids and vitamins than any other source of amino-acids. Flaxseed and hemp seeds are also excellent sources of amino acids. Amino acids are the building blocks of protein.

Renewed thinking: Protein is important in the right amount.

Action: I am eating only five to eight ounces of protein a day, balanced with vegetables. Or 1/3 of my body weight in grams; *if you weigh 125 lbs one third your weight is 41.66 so you average intake of protein should be around 41 to 45 grams a day.*

Sign and date:

PROTEIN AMOUNTS IN FOODS

Meats and fish - 4 ounces serving is equal to 30 grams

Quinoa - 1 cup is equal to six 6 grams

Organic eggs - 1 medium egg is equal to about 6 grams

Tuna fish - 3 ounces in water is equal to 18 grams

Hemp seeds - 1 cup is equal to about 60 grams

Raw nuts - 1 cup is equal to about 50-60 grams

Peanut butter or almond butter - 2 tablespoons equal to about 7 grams

Hummus - 2 tablespoons are equal to about 3 grams

Black beans - 1 cup is equal to about 7 grams

I endorse the consumption of organic wild caught foods whenever possible. This ensures that the fish, chicken, turkey or beef that you consume is not laden with chemicals, steroids, antibiotics or hormones. The animal grazes and eats grass, which builds its flesh into strong, healthy tissue with quality fats. In the case of diseased animals, studies show unsanitary, unhealthy housing conditions of animals are the problems. These conditions make it necessary for the grower to require antibiotics in the animal's food. These conditions exist for the convenience of the grower and the rapid weight gain of the animals.

The emphasis is on getting the animal fat so there is more weight when it is sold. Steroids with hormones for building muscle are also injected into the animals and can remain in the flesh until it is consumed. When we eat commercial animal foods, we could be and probably are consuming steroids meant for the growth of an animal, which definitely throws our body chemistry into an imbalanced state. It is better to not eat animals if you cannot find clean, farm-raised food.

As many health-supportive diets still include fish and eggs as protein sources, let me comment especially on them. Fish is a high-quality protein food that contains the fatty acids the body needs for proper brain function and hormone production. Psychological and emotional diseases and disorders have been treated with foods rich in Omega-3 fatty acids, which you can get from fish.

Fish should be wild or organic farm-raised. Farm-raised fish, fed synthetic chemicals and dyes have no beneficial oils. A good fish market will know the difference and will be glad to discuss it with you. The smaller fish are the least naturally polluted by the waters they live in. The water the fish live in has become the problem with fish. Eat only a small amount, two or three servings a week, if you are healthy. The healthy body should be able to eliminate the toxins that may be in the fish. Never eat the skin—fat is where the toxins are stored. Today we are seeing record amounts of mercury in fish so the smaller fish are cleaner and better to consume, if you are choosing fish. If you are pregnant you may want to be really cautious with fish and only eat very small fish like sardines.

As for eggs, they are a God-given food. They contain lecithin to help our bodies deal with the cholesterol that is also present. Eggs can be considered a very good protein source, but this is dependent upon the source of the egg, the care of the animal that laid the egg, and that it is cooked. Most commercially-fed chickens have very little Omega-3 fatty acids in their eggs because of the feed they're eating, so I would never consume eggs that are not organic in nature.

Organic eggs have the benefit of a concentrated protein and Omega-3 fatty acids that assist our brain development and help our body digest the protein in the eggs. Do not overcook eggs. Proteins become harder to digest, the longer the egg is cooked. A light scramble or a soft-boiled egg is the best way to consume cooked eggs.

Renewed thinking: There is a big difference between organic and nonorganic fish and eggs and between commercial animals raised by Amish or clean farming practices.

Action: I am easily finding a store that carries quality animal foods without added hormones or antibiotics, including organic eggs and wild or organic fish. I only consume organic protein sources.

Sign and date:

Cholesterol is a necessary substance in the body. If you don't consume cholesterol, your body will make it. Because high cholesterol is associated with heart disease, it is assumed that low blood cholesterol is good news, but recent research has proven this is not true. Low cholesterol levels are associated with strokes and low hormone production. Cholesterol is needed in the body to make hormones that control many different body and brain functions. It is a myth that eating foods high in cholesterol is the only cause of blockages and hardening of the arteries.

First of all, your body will manufacture cholesterol daily, based on the amount of cholesterol you consume. The less cholesterol you consume, the more your body produces. The rise in serum cholesterol levels comes from digesting and eating a high level of simple carbohydrate foods that convert quickly to sugar as well. Refined, processed foods cause artery damage that leads to the need for cholesterol. Sugar and refined foods like white breads, cakes and pastries, which have no vitamin and mineral content and no fiber left in them, cause inflammation that the body needs to repair.

Plaque that attaches itself to the artery walls is made up of many substances: fibrin, collagen, proteins and minerals that have drawn themselves out of synthetic, artificial, man-made fats (the partially hydrogenated vegetable oils we discussed).

Cholesterol is actually a plug or healing agent covering an irritation on the inside wall of the arteries. Yes, it can become a problem, but it is really trying to solve an already existing problem. This is why a total diet-makeover is necessary to produce a healthy body. Taking a drug that artificially lowers the tested numbers only causes a different problem somewhere else in the body.

The sooner you eliminate the processed and synthetic, artificial foods that cause the problems, the better health you will have. I understand it is sometimes necessary to take drugs, but this is a temporary intervention. Working with an aware, alternative health care professional can help you eventually eliminate medications, and the body will function when given health-supportive foods.

I am also aware this is a personal choice. The information provided in this book is for your consideration as well as to assist you in making a choice. My goal for you is to eat only whole, nutrient-dense vegetable-quality foods. The length of time and the process you choose are your choices alone. There is benefit to every little change you make.

Just eliminating one soda pop each day is equal to seventy-seven fewer teaspoons of sugar per week or 3.2 fewer pounds of sugar a month. I encourage immediate change and when you've adjusted to one change, go ahead and make the next change.

Eliminating three, quarter-pound hamburgers per week equals approximately two pounds of saturated fat each month. Then, walking just one-half mile three times a week is equal to six miles a month. Adding quality as you eliminate dead food is very important to a health supportive lifestyle. Each positive change you make will encourage you to make additional positive changes.

What is your long-term goal for yourself at this time? Keep the goal of being in a healthy body in front of you daily. Join a healthy body, a group of individuals pursuing health and wellbeing together at www.katwrightnd.com. Once you have signed up for the free support, you will get weekly messages and health updates about the latest information and tips for making healthy choices.

Every day tell yourself, I am in a healthy body

I want to acknowledge your commitment to read thus far and put in writing whatever you have so far committed to. Congratulations, you are an overcomer and a leader on the path of success at whatever you chose to be or do. I am leaving lots of room on the pages for your notes and opinions. Whatever you think is worth noting, write it down. I also leave room or margin in my life so there is always room for the unexpected. This is a great habit, but during some stages of life, it is difficult to find margin. Keep the idea in your mind and look for a daily time to block out when you can use it for yourself or others.

Give yourself room to rest, take a few extra deep breaths or if someone really needs you, then drop everything and help. If you'll leave room or margin, it does not put your life in turmoil when the unexpected shows up.

CHAPTER 13

COW'S MILK AGENDA

Cow's milk and refined sugar make two of the largest contributions to food-induced ill health in the United States. No wonder bone health is also one of the largest problems in the US. Milk is not a good food for bone health. If it were the prefect food for bone health why do we suffer from bone disease? We have dealt with refined sugar; now it is time to address the other staple of the Standard American Diet (SAD, remember?). There are other problems with milk products as the center of our diet. Its high protein content makes milk very acid-forming to our systems, which leads to organ and system breakdowns. I will say this; if you want to know more, you will have to dig deep because the dairy industry is big and has the power to cover the truth behind research and medical reports.

The truth is that homogenized milk is one of the major causes of heart disease in this country. Many doctors and dietitians know this truth, but will not deal with the issues because their professions are controlled and subsidized at the educational level by the dairy industry. It is grounds for losing your license if you do not follow protocol.

The dairy industry is trying to cover these issues by adding nutrients to milk that help aid in the digestion and absorption of calcium. This does not even begin to address the problem, much less solve it. The problem with milk products begins with modern breeding methods, which are designed to produce cows with abnormally large pituitary glands so that they produce three times more milk than the old-fashioned cow. Then these cows are fed high-protein, soy-based feeds instead of fresh green grass. As a result, they need antibiotics to keep them well. The antibiotics are found in the milk consumed by the public and we become resistant to antibiotics.

Milk also needs to be pasteurized and homogenized in order to sell it and ship it all over the country, let alone the world. When milk is pasteurized, all the valuable enzymes (lactase for the assimilation of lactose; galactase for the assimilation of galactose; phosphatase for the assimilation of calcium) are destroyed.

Without these enzymes, milk is impossible to digest properly. The human pancreas is not always able to produce these enzymes and overstress of the pancreas can lead to many diseases, with diabetes being the most obvious. Is it any wonder that diabetes is rampant and increasing in the United States?

When milk is homogenized, it breaks up its fat content into very small particles so they are evenly distributed. This fat in the blood is a hindrance to other beneficial nutrients and oxygen the body needs.

In the early forties, the Weston Price Institute published extensive research on the processed nature of homogenized and pasteurized milk and the degenerative effects of milk consumption. When the butterfat of commercial milk is homogenized, it is subject to rancidity. Even worse, butterfat may be removed altogether. Skim milk is sold as a health food, but the truth is that butterfat exists in milk for a reason. Without the fat, the body cannot absorb or utilize the vitamins and minerals in the milk. Synthetic vitamin D, known to be toxic to the liver, is added to replace the natural vitamin D complex in butterfat. Butterfat also contains natural acids that have strong anti-carcinogenic properties.

Nonfat dried milk is added to 1 percent and 2 percent milk. Cholesterol in fresh milk plays a variety of health promoting roles, but the cholesterol in nonfat dried milk is oxidized. In other words, it's rancid, and it is this rancid cholesterol that promotes heart disease.

This is not a quality food to be consumed on a regular basis. In fact, many people who think they could not do without milk actually have an allergy-relationship with dairy. It has been scientifically demonstrated that, when you are allergic to some foods, you crave them.

Cow's milk is the number one allergic food in this country. It has been well documented as a cause in diarrhea, cramps, bloating, gas, gastrointestinal bleeding, iron-deficiency, anemia, skin rashes, atherosclerosis and acne. I can tell you story after story of men and women who did not think they had a problem digesting milk products until they eliminated them from their diets and saw how much better they felt and how much weight they lost.

I even helped a man and woman, who wanted to start a family but could not get pregnant, understand that an allergy to dairy products could be their problem. They had both been tested for fertility and no problems were found, yet they could not conceive. Because milk and cheese were over 50 percent of their diets, they came to understand they could have a problem there, so they eliminated milk products from their diets. After giving their bodies three months to cleanse and adding more fresh vegetables and whole grains, the woman became pregnant and today has a healthy family of three children, all of whom are allergic to milk products just as she and her husband are.

One of the major problems with our modern-day milk has to do with a substance in the fat of the milk, called xanthine oxidase or XO, a protein enzyme. Medical research indicates that xanthine oxidase in the blood causes heart attacks by attacking the heart and arteries. When non-homogenized milk is consumed, XO is excreted like any other waste. But when milk is homogenized, the breakup of the fat allows tiny particles of XO to go through the walls of the intestine into the bloodstream and reach the heart and artery tissues, explains Dr. Kurt Oster, chief of cardiology at Park Hospital, Bridgeport, Connecticut. The XO acts chemically to scar the artery walls and heart tissue. The body tries to repair the damage by raising the cholesterol level of the blood and depositing protective fatty material on the scars. If the process continues, the material begins to clog the arteries, causing heart disease.

Heart disease is one of the single greatest causes of death in this country. Over one million Americans (1,054,500 to be exact) will die of heart disease and related diseases this year. Many cardiologist now will tell you, "The first thing I do with heart patients is take them off homogenized milk."

The recent approval (by the Federal Drug Administration) of the use of Bovine Growth Hormone (BGH), by dairy farmers to increase their milk production, only makes milk more dangerous to Americans' health. BGH increases milk production by cows and also causes an increase in an insulin-like growth factor (IGF-1) in the milk of treated cows. IGF-1 survives milk pasteurization and human intestinal digestion. It can be directly absorbed into the human bloodstream, particularly in infants.

Medical research shows it is possible that IGF-1 promotes the transformation of human breast cells to cancerous forms. IGF-1 is also a growth factor for already cancerous breast and colon cancer cells, promoting their progression and invasiveness. It is also possible for us to absorb the BGH directly from the milk we drink or from any product made from milk. This will cause further IGF-1 production by our own cells.

BGH also decreases the body fat of cows, which is already contaminated with a wide range of carcinogens, pesticides, dioxin and antibiotic residues from the feed. Because body fat holds toxins, when cows have less body fat, these toxic substances are then transported into the cow's milk.

On top of health problems this new growth hormone is creating, take a look at the financial problems it will cause our country. More milk from the big producers means more farmers will be put out of business. More milk means additional subsidization from Uncle Sam, to the tune of $65 million in 1994 and $116 million in 1995. The Office of Management and Budget (OMB) predicts it will cost Americans $300 million to $500 million over the next six years in additional price supports to milk farmers.

I also feel the need to address milk as a raw food.

It may be consumed in a health-supportive diet and it does contain the enzymes that are necessary to aid in digestion. But let me caution you. In America, we consume so much dairy that to substitute the raw milk for the altercated, homogenized, processed stuff is a good step but *only* a step. High dairy consumption in the past will still cause problems with digestion if the dairy consumption is not stopped for a number of years. The body needs time to eliminate the consequences of a high dairy consumption diet. Dairy consumed as a fermented food occasionally may not cause problems for a healthy body. There is much controversy over this topic. It is important that cows are grass-fed and the dairy product is kept sterile and clean **without the addition of bleach**. Then, for the digestion to be comfortable, it should be fermented into yogurt or soft cheese like blue cheese or feta. In addition, this is only an occasional part of the diet.

Despite the consumption of dairy foods, which are famous for their rich sources of calcium, there has been a widespread calcium deficiency in the United States for more than two hundred years. We are a nation of calcium-deficient diseases, yet we continue to tell people to drink their milk. If milk is the solution to the calcium issue, why do we have a calcium deficiency epidemic? The truth is that we are not deficient in calcium. We are simply unable to absorb the calcium we consume.

Milk is not a good source of absorbable calcium. Its calcium is bound by phosphorus, as well as in poor balance with magnesium and potassium, which are necessary for calcium absorption, so only 20 to 30 percent of the calcium in milk is usable by the body. Milk protein also accelerates calcium excretion from the blood through the kidneys. The issue is not only how much calcium is consumed but rather how many other things in the diet interfere with the calcium absorption, or put a higher demand on calcium needs.

Many, many factors increase the need for calcium: soft drinks, sugar, high protein foods, alcohol, caffeine, some drugs and foods high in oxalic acid (like potatoes, tomatoes, and cooked spinach). Elimination of these problem foods and the addition of magnesium, phosphorus and vitamins D and K have been proven over and over to help with the problem of calcium deficiency.

You will see much more about vitamin D in the news soon. Do you know we did not even have a test to check blood levels of vitamin D until 1997? There has been much revealing new information about vitamin D. The system our bodies use to make vitamin D is one that we go out into the sun and make thousands of units of cholecalciferol, which the liver then turns into 25(OH). Our organs then make a steroid hormone called 1, 25-D, which helps regulate genes in every organ of the body. One of those important functions is calcium absorption.

We need to think about this for a minute, since science now tells us it takes twenty minutes of full body exposure to make the amount of 1, 25-D our bodies need each day.

We can get Vitamin K, magnesium and phosphorus from our foods, but what about the vitamin D? On top of the fact that we do not have the time in the middle of the day (in our culture) to get that sun exposure, we have actually been told to cover up and hide from the sun. For the sake of staying on the calcium topic, does it make any sense to keep upping calcium without getting vitamin D? It may seem impossible to get enough calcium rich foods into the diet, but that is because we are used to processed fast foods, and we are not getting results by just adding calcium supplements. Instead of using homogenized, processed products as our calcium source, we could think of these foods as the poisons they are and avoid them as if our lives depend on it, because they do. I have not consumed homogenized, pasteurized cow's milk products for over thirty years.

The milk I did consume for a time was raw milk and I found, as research shows, even though it has enzymes to assist in digestion, it is a stress at the least on our digestive systems. If you have any digestive problems, arthritis or skin issues, even though there may be slight benefit to some to consume these cow milk foods, you should eliminate even raw cow's milk products from your diet. Research points out to us the addictive nature of cow's milk sugar and fat. The only way you will know is to eliminate this food for at least three months. If it is the only thing you eliminate, you may not see the results I am expecting. This can be a stubborn addiction.

Renewed thinking: Dairy products in this country are a problem.

Action: I am reducing my consumption of dairy with the goal to eliminate this processed food.

Sign and date:

Current research is looking at the importance of vitamin D in overall health and immune strength.

This is an important topic for Americans who, today, are the true cavemen and women. We leave our homes from the garage before the sun comes up for many. We park in garages while we work in buildings where there is no sun exposure. Calcium absorption and immune function have been proven to be dependent on sufficient vitamin D. UVB exposure on the skin causes the skin to produce Vitamin D, but UVA exposure actually destroys Vitamin D. When you are outside in the sun, the body will make vitamin D in amounts it needs, but when you are riding in your car or getting sun exposure through glass, the only UV rays you are getting are the damaging UVA.

Researchers are saying it actually takes one hour of full body exposure every day to get adequate vitamin D. On top of that, while the vitamin D is on the skin it is not totally absorbed for up to twenty-four hours. So do not shower with soap after you are in the sun for the maximum benefit of vitamin D for at least twenty-four hours. On top of these modern-day issues to our health a precursor to vitamin D production is cholesterol.

If you are taking drugs to lower cholesterol, this in turn decreases your body's vitamin D levels as well. It may seem confusing, but one thing many of the health-conscious individuals I know are doing is supplementing with vitamin D and seeing major improvements in health issues, from blood sugar regulation and insulin uptake to hormone functions. Taking an oral sublingual vitamin D3 eliminates the whole issue of absorbing the vitamin D3 from your skin. However, be aware that any time you use oral vitamin D, you will want to have your levels checked regularly using a qualified lab such as LabCorp, to make sure you are within optimal range and avoid overdosing.

The important point here is to have your vitamin D levels checked.

Why is vitamin D associated with preventing so many different diseases from breast cancer to skin disease and many other health benefits? Let me answer that for you. Dr. John Cannel, MD, has done extensive research on this topic and lectures at medical conventions nationwide.

Understanding the basic science of vitamin D is important to understand why this substance prevents so many conditions. Vitamin D is not found in the human diet. It is a substrate or precursor for a powerful steroid hormone the body makes and is involved in multiple functions in the body. Steroid hormones turn on specific genes, depending on the hormone.

The steroid hormone the body produces from Vitamin D is responsible for regulating or building over two thousand genes. That means over two-thousand mechanisms of action on different enzymes are responsible for the immune function in the body.

The best form of vitamin D comes from the sun, but the fear created by skin cancer caused by sun exposure has kept Americans out of the sun. The epidemics created by vitamin D deficiency have increased because of the past twenty years of dermatological recommendations to avoid the sun. It is true that overexposure to UV rays is harmful, but the vitamin D we need is made in thirty minutes of full body exposure. After that, the sunblock can be applied and the levels of sun exposure controlled. If you have thirty minutes of full sun where you live and if you have the time in the middle of the day when the sun is at its strongest, full body exposure would provide you with optimal levels of vitamin D. The other option is oral supplements. Oral supplements are the easiest choice. Most African Americans need longer exposure to the sun to make the vitamin D they need, and most adults do not have the time needed every day to exposure themselves to the sun. Google vitamin D and see how many reports are published daily on this important health topic.

Even though you may or may not have heard or read, vitamin D is good for three serious epidemics in the United States with children. These out-of-control and ever-increasing diseases are type 1 diabetes (auto immune disease), asthma, and autism. These conditions have proven to be directly related to the deficiency of vitamin D in a pregnant woman.

The Canadian Pediatric Society has increased the vitamin D recommendation for pregnant women up to 2000 mg a day and some researchers recommend that pregnant women get 5000 mg of vitamin D daily. Research has shown that vitamin D begins to be stored in the body after the blood levels go over 50 mg/ml. You must have a lab test after two to four months of taking a vitamin D supplement, because oral vitamin D is not the natural way to get this vitamin. Your levels should be over forty and close to seventy for what the researches are seeing at this time.

The important thing to note is the experts in the study of vitamin D think we will even see a need for more. Right now, it is important to see how your body absorbs this important vitamin because we are all different. You may choose to wait until this information reaches the main stream of information or do you homework and understand why all the researchers and their family and friends are supplementing with the vitamin right now because of the huge value they are seeing.

You are successful the moment you start moving towards a worthwhile goal.

You have to think about the big things while doing the small things so all the small things go in the right direction.

See yourself healthy and transformed into the person you would like to be with the health you would like to have.

You are changing your basic belief system about food as you progress through this book. Stay on track and finish with Your Health.

Nobody can go back and start a new beginning but anyone can start today and create a new ending
        - Maria Robinson

CHAPTER 14

NUTRIENTS

This is an overview of the nutrients we need and how to absorb them from our foods

Protein is found in:

- ❖ Animal flesh
- ❖ Fish flesh
- ❖ Soybeans (although I do not recommend eating much)
- ❖ Legumes (beans)
- ❖ Seeds—hemp and flax
- ❖ Raw organic dairy (only eat this type of dairy)
- ❖ Nuts
- ❖ Rye flour
- ❖ Quinoa
- ❖ Millet
- ❖ Amaranth
- ❖ Okra
- ❖ Watercress
- ❖ Yams
- ❖ Spirulina
- ❖ Barley grass
- ❖ Bee pollen
- ❖ Nutritional yeast or brewer's yeast

Enzyme nutrients needed for absorption are hydrochloric acid (HCL) and protease. These enzymes are made in the body, but as we age we usually make less. They can be supplemented and help relieve deficiency symptoms.

Protein deficiency symptoms:
- ❖ Temporomandibular joint pain (TMJ)
- ❖ Edema
- ❖ Slow wound-healing
- ❖ High blood pressure
- ❖ Hormone imbalance
- ❖ Constant hunger
- ❖ Depression
- ❖ Unhealthy hair, skin, or nails
- ❖ Maintaining pH of the blood
- ❖ Energy
- ❖ Cold hands and feet
- ❖ Craving for crunchy, salty foods
- ❖ Difficulty losing weight
- ❖ Increased watery secretions (may even spit while speaking)

Protein balance is easily obtained from a vegetarian diet, if you eat a diet high in vegetables, seeds, nuts and whole grains. It may not be your desire to consume a complete vegetable diet, but whatever you choose, it is important to eat adequate protein and to digest it. You could be presenting a deficiency even if you eat enough protein, if you do not digest it. This is where we see the importance of HCL and protease. Overcooking protein-rich foods makes them resistant to enzyme action in the digestive tract.

When you think of carbohydrates, you should realize there are different kinds of carbohydrates. There are the ones I have spoken of already, that you want to avoid in the processed, refined, dead foods, while there are other carbohydrates we want to consume.

The simple carbohydrates feed yeast overgrowth and lead to empty calories.

Quality carbohydrates are found in:
- ❖ Vegetables
- ❖ Whole grains
- ❖ Potatoes and other root vegetables
- ❖ Brown rice and vegetables
- ❖ Seeds and nuts

The enzymes needed to digest carbohydrates are:
- ❖ Salivary and pancreatic enzymes containing amylase
- ❖ Carbohydrase
- ❖ Suctrase
- ❖ Maltase
- ❖ Glycoamylase
- ❖ Galactose

Enzyme deficiency symptoms:
- ❖ The person startles easily
- ❖ Voice becomes high pitched under stress
- ❖ Mouth sores
- ❖ Muscle weakness
- ❖ Frequently irritated throat
- ❖ Inability to relax
- ❖ Dry conditions in the body (eyes, mouth and nose)
- ❖ Tenderness in the salivary glands (rub under the chin on either side of the tongue)
- ❖ Dry stools
- ❖ Constipation

It is very important to mention that excess carbohydrates are stored as fat in the body. **If you do not digest what you eat, it is stored as toxins and fat, reducing the oxygen flow to organs and can cause disease.**

Trace minerals are extremely important as well. I prefer to get the bulk of the nutrition needed from foods.

Sources of trace minerals:
- ❖ Root vegetables
- ❖ Honey
- ❖ Black strap molasses
- ❖ Whole grains
- ❖ Nuts
- ❖ Meat
- ❖ Sea vegetables
- ❖ Alfalfa
- ❖ Dandelion
- ❖ Kelp
- ❖ Sage
- ❖ Rose hips
- ❖ Celtic sea salt
- ❖ Himalayan sea salt

Mineral deficiency symptoms:
- ❖ Vertigo
- ❖ Chemical imbalance
- ❖ General fatigue
- ❖ Excessive thirst, that cannot be relieved
- ❖ Electrolyte imbalance

Vitamin E is found in
- ❖ Sunflower seeds
- ❖ Almonds
- ❖ Olives
- ❖ Papaya
- ❖ Avocados

- ❖ Hazelnuts
- ❖ Turnip greens
- ❖ Bean sprouts
- ❖ Egg yokes
- ❖ Alfalfa
- ❖ Bee pollen
- ❖ Kelp
- ❖ Rose hips

Vitamin E deficiency symptoms:

- ❖ Heart conditions
- ❖ Lack of energy
- ❖ Poor circulation
- ❖ PMS, fluid retention, tender breast
- ❖ Asthma
- ❖ Scarring
- ❖ Tingling or loss of sensation in hands and feet

Vitamin E is best obtained from foods. If you do supplement Vitamin E, there are some things you need to know about supplements. Whole-form vitamin E is the most beneficial. To be whole, it must contain d-alpha, beta, delta and gamma tocopherols, as well as alpha, beta, delta and gamma tocotrienols. If the bottle says only one or part of these, it is not whole and if the bottle says "dl" before the alpha, beta, delta and gamma, it is a synthetic vitamin. Do not take it. Vitamin E acetate is also synthetic. Do not consume it orally or use it on your skin topically.

Vitamin E occurs naturally, along with amino acids and phospholipids that make it effective as a food or a topical cream or serum. There has been conflicting research on vitamin E and the problem lies in the type of vitamin used. Synthetic vitamins are not the same as a whole food, even if they are synthesized from whole foods.

Balancing blood sugar levels in the body is one of the most important factors in maintaining proper energy and weight. What we eat, the quality of food and how it is prepared, affects the release of energy or the sugar level in the blood. Balancing protein, carbohydrates, and foods containing vitamin minerals and trace mineral will balance our health.

Eating nutrient-dense whole natural foods at every meal and avoiding simple sugars and carbohydrates as well as coffee and soda will allow the body to comfortably regulate the blood sugar levels.

If blood sugar goes too low, we experience fatigue, poor concentration, irritability, headache and even digestive problems that lead to premature aging.

High blood sugar levels damage arteries, making them less receptive to insulin, which helps cells receive sugar and use it as energy. High blood sugar requires more insulin, but if the damaged cell walls are not receptive to insulin, the body keeps making more and the sugar is turned into fat, leading to a cycle of weight gain, damage and eventually disease.

To keep the blood sugar levels balanced, eat complex carbohydrates like vegetables and grain, along with quality proteins like beans, nuts and low-fat animal proteins; avoiding simple carbohydrates like cakes, cookies, candies, soft drinks, coffee and other quick-energy drinks and foods.

Inflammation causing premature aging in the form of damage to arteries, joints and even brain tissue occurs when certain chemicals are consumed or just as a result of the use of much needed oxygen. Antioxidants stop this damage. They are the equivalent to a fire extinguisher in the body.

An easy way to boost your antioxidant consumption is to add fresh berries and seeds or nuts to your breakfast, as well as to consume them as mid-day snacks. By having a fresh salad and a side dish of lightly cooked vegetables, you also add antioxidants to your daily diet.

Homocysteine is a type of protein found in the blood that is naturally turned into to beneficial chemicals in a healthy body. The body's most important antioxidant, glutathione

(and another very important nutrient to both the body and brain called SAMe), assists in the production of important chemical reactions in the body. However, without optimal nutrition, especially the necessary B vitamins, homocysteine can accumulate and increase the risk of over fifty different diseases. Once again we see how important it is to consume nutrient-rich foods.

Homocysteine levels are the one factor that medical professionals say can determine if you will live a long life. Homocysteine is a protein produced by the body and found in the blood. Ideally homocysteine levels should be low. Homocysteine is made from an amino acid (methionine) found in dietary protein. Homocysteine levels are important in the diagnosis of heart disease and the body's overall health. The body uses homocysteine to make two very important antioxidants—glutathione and SAMe.

Research has shown us that *antioxidants work together to form a network that fights damage and keeps cells strong*. Glutathione is the key antioxidant in the network. All other antioxidants work together to raise the intracellular levels of glutathione, the most important in the antioxidant network defense system. The body makes glutathione from the other nutrients. The glutathione levels can measure the body's overall levels of antioxidants.

SAMe is what is called (in medical terms) a methyl donor. The ability of the body to maintain a chemical balance necessary at all times is dependent on its ability to subtract and add necessary molecules that create the chemicals and hormones needed at any given moment. The adding and subtracting of a methyl group occurs billions of times every second, within the body, keeping everything in balance.

If levels of B vitamins in the body are deficient, homocysteine cannot be converted. As homocysteine levels raise, damage to arteries, brain and DNA occur. This is an important indicator of the risk of heart disease, cancer and Alzheimer's, as well as the body's ability to adjust and adapt to daily stress and activity.

A good quality vitamin and mineral supplement should always contain B2, 6, 12, folic acid, trimethyl glycine (TMJ) and zinc to assist the body with its important functions. Nutrient-dense foods that contain vitamins, minerals and trace elements (needed to assimilate foods into chemicals that can be biologically used in the daily functions of the body) are essential.

I mention this important often-overlooked test to be added to your blood pressure, cholesterol and weight measurements. Homocysteine is the very best indicator of your future health and, if the levels are high, it is one more reason you may choose to change to a nutrient-dense whole foods diet.

Phyto-chemicals are micronutrients found in fresh foods, but because they are not vitamins or minerals, our lives do not directly depend on them. They do, however, assist other key nutrients, antioxidants and hormones to perform their roles of promoting health and preventing disease.

Phyto-chemicals are not stored in the body; therefore, they need to be consumed regularly. Hundreds of phyto-chemicals have been identified and are easy to add to the diet.

> **Allium compounds** found in garlic, onions, chives and shallots are shown to block the conversion of nitrates into cancer-causing nitrosamines, as well as slowing the action of aflatoxins (cancer-causing agents found in rancid foods, especially peanuts and soy) found in peanuts and other foods. Allium-containing foods have the reputation as preventive to stomach and colon cancer. Garlic is reported to significantly lower cholesterol and help prevent blood clots.

> **Bioflavonoids** are found in rosehips, citrus fruit, berries, broccoli, cherries, melon, plums, tea, tomatoes and red wine. They help detoxify heavy metals in the body, stabilize vitamin C and support capillary strength to protect against bleeding gums, varicose veins, hemorrhoids, strains and bruises.

> **Chlorophyll** found in dark green plants has been shown to protect against cancer and support red blood cell strength and production in bone marrow. A great source of chlorophyll is grasses grown from cereal grains that are gluten free for those individuals who are gluten sensitive or with celiac disease.

Ellagic acids metabolize carcinogens before they can damage DNA. They are found in strawberries, grapes and raspberries. Studies show that strawberries and raspberries stop nitrosamine, a cancer-causing chemical found in meat, because of their ellagic acid content.

Glucosinolates are one of the most important anti-cancer nutrients because of their supportive role in detoxifying the liver. The World Cancer Research Fund stated that there is evidence that foods high in glucosinolates such as broccoli, broccolini, and Brussels sprouts reduce the risk of lung, stomach, colorectal and probably breast cancers.

The doors we open and close each day decide the life we live.
        - Flora Whittemore

CHAPTER 15

ADDITIVES AND GM FOODS

I prefer to focus on what you need to do to support health, but I would be remiss if I did not address food additives and Genetically Modified (GM) foods. If you eat the typical American diet, you probably consume more than five thousand different synthetic chemicals in your daily diet and more than six pounds of preservatives and artificial chemical compounds each year. These ingredients are sources of damaging free radicals that cause a host of diseases and prematurely age the body. The needed research on GM's has not been done and we are eating this food anyway and don't know it.

A high-protein diet and the combination of over two thousand five hundred chemical additives are the formula for cancer and degenerative disease. Additives get into our food by way of many disguises and under many different names. They may be called colorings, flavorings, stabilizers, solidifiers, preservatives or emulsifiers. There is one thing they all have in common—

They are destroyers of our health.

Dr. Ben Feingold has done a tremendous service to mankind. Through many hours of research, he has found that hyperkinetic children can be brought under control simply by changing some of their food habits and eliminating additives from their diets. This additive-free diet has changed children who were previously acting like animals, back to loving, easy-to-live-with youngsters. This way of life has been a real blessing to many families.

Probably the most consumed "treat" in America is the one most filled with chemical additives. What would a party be without ice cream? Are you aware that at least one hundred chemicals can be added to ice creams that do not have to be put on the label?

Below are a few of the most common preservatives. All those **not** listed have the same problems associated with their consumption. I do not eat foods that *need* or *have* additives.

BHA and BHT are preservatives added to dry cereals to prevent hydrogenated vegetable oil from going rancid. Experiments in Australia found that when rats were fed BHA/BHT, their blood cholesterol went sky high and their hair fell out. But of more importance, some of the offspring born to rats that ate the same amount of BHA/BHT (proportionate to what is found in our food), were born with no eyes.

TARTRAZINE OR E102 is a food coloring known to cause hyperactivity and allergies in sensitive children.

CALCIUM SULFATE is nothing more than plaster of Paris. It is great for patching cracks in a wall—and for making it easier to knead five-hundred-pound batches of dough in giant machines. It is not good for you at all, but it makes better imitation bread.

BLUE NO. 1 is used in baked goods, dessert mixes, ice cream, dietary supplements and candy. It causes allergic reactions and malignant tumors in rats.

CITRUS RED NO.2 is used to mask the greenness that oranges have. This dye has been shown to have carcinogenic activity. Because the dye does not penetrate the peel, treated oranges are probably safe, so long as the peel is not eaten and you wash the orange before and after removing the peel. Be sure to also wash your hands to remove any residual dye.

ORANGE B is used to color frankfurter and sausage casings. It is chemically related to Red No.2. Allergies, even though they may not typically consider the source a food additive, may occur and could be related to orange B in foods.

YELLOW NO. 5 is used in butter, margarine and candies. It can cause wheezing, asthmatic symptoms and hives. It is carcinogenic when tested on rats.

MSG (monosodium glutamate) is used as a food flavoring, but what it actually does is irritate the wall of the stomach to a stage of bright red, acute congestion. This acute congestion causes a hunger sensation so that you ask for a second helping. Acute congestion of the stomach is an almost ideal way to cause cancer.

MSG also irritates the thyroid gland and speeds up heart rate. MSG attaches itself to the numerous glutamate receptors within your heart's electrical conduction system and the heart muscle itself. Therefore it can be damaging to your heart. It may even explain the sudden deaths sometimes seen among young athletes. Research abounds, showing that MSG may lead to obesity, eye damage, headaches, fatigue, depression and a host of other negative symptoms. It is a damaging brain stimulant referred to as excitotoxins (chemicals that immediately excite the brain and cause oxidative damage to the brain, killing brain cells) by Dr. Russell Blaylock in his extensive essay on the subject, "Health and Nutrition Secrets that Can Save Your Life!" This extensive work describes how MSG leads to massive free-radical damage to the body and the brain.

The following ingredients may contain MSG along with other additives I consider toxins: autolyzed yeast, glutamate, monopotassium glutamate, textured protein, yeast nutrient, calcium caseinate, glutamic acid, monosodium glutamate, gelatin, hydrolyzed protein, sodium caseinate, flavors, flavorings, natural chicken flavoring, stock, enzyme modified, protease, seasonings, broth carrageena, corn starch, pasteurized soy sauce, soy protein isolate, malt extract, lacto-dextrin, pectin, powered milk, beef flavoring, bouillon, and barley malt.

Generally, processed foods that contain these products have an ingredient list that is as long and incomprehensible as the list above. When I see an ingredient list like this, I don't bother reading it. I know I do not want to consume that which is not truly food.

Aspartame is the technical name for the brand names NutraSweet, Equal, Spoonful and Equal-Measure. It is also one of the most dangerous chemicals that should never have been allowed to be added into food. Products containing aspartame are sold in over a hundred countries and are consumed by over 250 million people worldwide. At the end of 2008, aspartame was found in over 6,000 products—everything from soft drinks to frozen desserts, yogurt and chewable vitamins.

The agencies that are supposed to protect you and teach you about nutritional needs have vested financial interests in maintaining the belief that aspartame is safe. Loads of money and political careers are at stake if this scam is revealed. Do not expect the major news and medical industries to cut off the hand that feeds them. Come to understand this about the business of health.

The approval process for aspartame was one of scandal, bribes and other shady practices within the pharmaceutical industry, large American corporations and even the FDA. I am sure you are not surprised to hear this, but why do we turn to them for the truth? Initially, the FDA actually denied the approval of aspartame, due to flawed data, brain tumor findings in animal studies and lack of studies on humans to determine longer-term effects.

Unfortunately, despite these valid concerns, including evidence of its neurotoxicity, aspartame was successfully pushed through to the market. You guessed it, financial promises and power shifts brought about the approval of this toxic chemical as a food. Test subjects in studies that were not tainted by conflict of interest, did indeed suffer health problems.

It boggles my mind to try to understand how any educated person could come to the conclusion that this is a safe food in the face of available evidence spanning more than twenty-five years. I expect the governing food regulators to be cautious on the side of safety until all evidence is in, but it has proven the power of the money is greater than the concern for the health of the individual.

The European Food Safety Authority claims that the 2005 study by the Ramazzini Foundation (which concluded that aspartame causes significant increases in lymphomas/leukemia, and is a multi-potential carcinogen) was "deficient." It even dismissed the second study, performed by the same team in 2007, which showed that the aspartame-exposed rats developed so much formaldehyde in their bodies that their skin turned yellow. It is the formation of formaldehyde that is the link between aspartame and lymphoma and leukemia.

It is well known that aspartame turns into wood alcohol when it is consumed. However, what few people realize is that wood alcohol morphs into formaldehyde (the same stuff used for embalming) in the cells of your body.

Formaldehyde is a Class 1, cancer-causing agent, responsible for everything from sick-house syndrome to birth defects, and research shows it causes lymphoma and leukemia in both lab rats and humans.

The U.S. Environmental Protection Agency (EPA) listed formaldehyde as a "probable human carcinogen" as far back as 1987. In 2004, the International Agency for Research on Cancer classified it as a "known human carcinogen" based partly on available research linking it to leukemia. Aspartame intake has also been shown to increase the risk of breast and prostate cancer. Incidents of both types of cancer have been on the rise at a pace closely associated with the expanding use of aspartame throughout the world.

There are over nine hundred published studies on the health hazards of aspartame. (You can find a list in the National Library Medicine Index.) Formaldehyde created by aspartame accumulates in your body. As recently as May of 2009, the *Journal of the National Cancer Institute* published yet another study confirming the link between formaldehyde exposure and a significantly increased risk of dying from cancers of the blood and lymphatic system.

Industry mouthpieces claim that your body can quickly eliminate the formaldehyde formed by aspartame consumption, but previous research again claims otherwise. According to a 1998 study in *Life Sciences*, formaldehyde derived from dietary aspartame binds to tissues and accumulates in various organs, such as your liver, brown and white adipose tissues, muscle, brain, cornea, and retina.

The researchers stated:

"…regular intake of aspartame may result in the progressive accumulation of formaldehyde adducts. It may be further speculated that the formation of adducts can help to explain the chronic effects aspartame consumption may induce on sensitive tissue such as the brain. "

"In any case, the possible negative effects that the accumulation of formaldehyde adducts can induce is, obviously, long-term." "The alteration of protein integrity and function may need some time to induce substantial effects. The damage to nucleic acids, mainly to DNA may eventually induce cell death and/ or mutations." "…It is concluded that aspartame consumption may constitute a hazard because of its contribution to the formation of formaldehyde adducts."

Health problems initially reported included:
Neurological/behavioral symptoms(67 percent),including headaches, dizziness and mood changes, such as depression; gastrointestinal symptoms (24 percent); allergic type and/or dermatologic symptoms (15 percent); alterations in menstrual patterns (6 percent); other symptoms of various types (9 percent).

Today, there are some ten thousand documented reports of adverse reactions to aspartame, including death. But since it is estimated that only about 1 percent of people who experience a reaction report it, it is safe to assume at least a million people have had a reaction to this chemical.

Migraines are by far the most frequently reported reaction. You might not realize you're having a reaction to aspartame. In fact, most people don't make the connection and a tremendous amount of time and money is spent by aspartame "reactors" (people sensitive to the chemical) trying to find out why they are sick.

I can't overstate the importance of avoiding aspartame to protect your short and long-term health, the quality of your life and the lives of your loved ones. I hope you'll take this information to heart and eliminate aspartame and other artificial sweeteners from your diet.

Renewed thinking: I can eat without consuming food additives.

Now for the GM foods: This is the most recent and surprising lack of integrity we have experienced as consumers in America. Unlike safety evaluations for drugs, (even

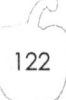

though this is a political joke) there are no human clinical trials of Genetically Modified (GM) foods. The only published human experiment revealed that the genetic material inserted into GM soy transfers into bacteria living inside our intestines that continues to function. This means that long after we stop eating GM foods, we may still have their GM proteins produced continuously inside us. At best we can only say the verdict is not in, but we do know someone stands to make a lot of money and gain a lot of control by genetically modifying seeds.

Pregnant mothers eating GM foods may endanger offspring. The food and drug administration is not protecting us like most of us think they are. They say the verdict is still out on the subject. If the verdict is not in yet, I chose to be safe and not sorry; as we have been with so many other food and drug situations.

The first and alarming problem is that embryo development can be adversely affected by tiny amounts of substances in the mother's diet, so with GM foods this could be a serious problem. GMs may alter gene expression in children of pregnant women and be passed on to future generations. Genetically Modified crops may contain substances that impact normal fetal development, but have never been adequately tested for these effects. If there is not adequate testing I would want to know as a pregnant consumer. Don't you?

GM foods are more dangerous for children than adults because children are generally more susceptible to toxins, allergens and nutritional problems due to their body weight

Children usually consume more milk which may be from cows treated with rbGH, (more about this in the milk chapter) and the emergence of antibiotic-resistant diseases may also significantly impact those children who are prone to recurring infections.

Action: I will read labels and reject whatever is enriched or preserved with food additives or genetically modified.

Sign and date:

You have the power to be part of the solution. For more information and to stop the insanity, take a look at the web site responsibletechnology.org

Patience and perseverance have a magical effect before which difficulties disappear and obstacles vanish. A little knowledge that acts is worth infinitely more than much knowledge that is idle.

- John Quincy Adams

CHAPTER 16

KNOWLEDGE IS OPPORTUNITY

Providing your body with essential nutrients every day, through a healthy combination of fresh vegetables, whole grains, low fat proteins, good quality fats, good calcium sources and fresh fruits is the first step in creating a healthier you. These foods will provide you with the antioxidants, vitamins and minerals you need to stay healthy and fight off the diseases of our developed country.

However, making changes in your diet and your lifestyle is very challenging and requires a great amount of dedication. It is also advantageous to have the support and encouragement of people who understand the importance of making a commitment to achieving better health. Ask others in your community to join you and transform their lives as well. In this way, you will become a part of a network of people making a difference for yourself and your children and friends.

The commitments you made in the beginning of the book will take you in the direction of success. In the next section, I will give you a specific plan you may choose to follow to help you start. Some people like to follow a recipe, and others just need some principles. Whichever you are, I am committed to your success and will leave you with the tools you need to succeed. My book *Your Health in Your Hands* is a cookbook with all the recipes you will ever need. You can also sign up for my video library of cooking shows at www. katwrightnd.com

I continue to remind you of the basics because with the basics you build your foundation of health.

The secret to your health, both mind and body is not to mourn the past or worry about the future but to live in the moment wisely and earnestly.

Use the knowledge you are gaining to live wisely.

Renewed thinking: I am able to make choices that will support my health.

Action: Starting now I will choose fresh vegetables, nuts and whole grains as the basis of my diet.

Sign and date:

The knowledge you need to make responsible choices is available.

CHAPTER 17

TOP TEN FOODS

GREEN FOODS

The American diet is primarily acid-forming, so adding green foods brings a much-needed alkaline aspect to the body. Green plant foods can be in the form of a green drink, fresh salad, or cooked side dish. If I had to pick a top green, it would be kale. It is versatile. It can be eaten cooked, raw, or juiced. Kale is high in antioxidants and has the highest-ranking oxygen-radical absorbance capacity (ORAC) of any of the green foods. (The U.S. Department of Agriculture applies the ORAC rating based on all the antioxidants in a food and the ability of the different antioxidants to work together as a team to fight free radicals.) In addition, kale's detoxifying enzymes may fight cancer and other chemicals that may cause cellular damage. Other greens in this category include the cabbage family foods, which are very high in cancer-fighting properties (broccoli, Brussels sprouts, collard greens, dandelion greens and dark green leafy lettuce).

The green foods category includes cereal grasses like barley and wheatgrass. It is easy to obtain cereal grasses. Usually every town has a juice bar serving up fresh wheatgrass shots. If not, you can always purchase from a variety of top-quality brands of powdered beverage mix containing cereal grasses.

Green cereal grasses are high in chlorophyll, which helps clean the lymphatic system and assist the blood. They are also rich in vitamins, phytonutrients and minerals. Each variety of grass contains a different, outstanding nutrient, which is why I like to consume a drink that combines many different grasses and sea vegetables. I find it the easiest and healthiest thing you can add to your lifestyle. An important note: do not try to grow your own microalgae.

There are growing conditions in which microalgae can be toxic, but if it is harvested properly this is not a problem.

NUTS AND SEEDS

Nut-and-seed eaters are recorded as having fewer heart attacks and less cancer. Nuts and seeds have Omega-3 and Omega-6 oils and are high in minerals, protein and fiber. A delicious variety of healthy dishes can be created using nuts and seeds as the base. Walnuts are my favorite nut because of the high quality Omega-3 fats and their delicious taste. Considered brain food, they contain protein, fiber, calcium, magnesium, phosphorus and potassium in a good balance and are beneficial throughout life for cognitive brain health, reproduction and growth to a mature adult. Other good nuts are almonds, hazelnuts, cashews, pine nuts, macadamia nuts, pecans and pistachios.

My favorite seed is the hemp seed because of its nutrient profile, simplicity and taste. Hemp is also a great protein source weighing in at 25 percent protein content. I use the tiny hemp seeds in a morning breakfast shake and on all my fresh salads. Hemp is rich in minerals, calcium, potassium, magnesium, sulfur and calcium. I put quinoa in this category. It is one of my top ten foods. People think it is a grain, but in reality it is a seed that acts like a grain. I eat it to keep from wanting other carbohydrate foods that are less nutritious. Combined with vegetables or in a salad and pilaf, it is a tasty, nutritious, filling and well-balanced food.

COLD-WATER FISH

Salmon and sardines are my favorites in the fish category. They are high in Omega-3 and, of course, protein, as well as easy to obtain if eating out or traveling. The type of Omega-3 oil differs in fish or nuts and seeds. Research shows that the Omega-3 in fish provides the cardiovascular benefits involved with EPA and DHA. The third kind of Omega-3 found in walnuts, flax seeds and the hemp seed is called ALA, which the body uses to make EPA and DHA.

I do limit the consumption of fish to no more than twice a week because of the potential mercury content. However, if kept healthy, the body can naturally eliminate this toxin and the consumption of the fish can be very beneficial, especially when not at home, as a protein source. Sea vegetables, especially chlorella, can help eliminate mercury along with other toxic metals. This category can be satisfied by taking a krill oil supplement as well. Krill are the small fish that the larger fish feed on. They are smaller and so do not have the toxic levels of mercury contained in the larger fish.

SPROUTS

Eating small plants keeps the body hydrated and nourished. Research done on these tiny plants called sprouts reveals significant cancer-reducing properties and a powerhouse of nutrients. I love the crunch, and they are a complete package. I especially love lentil sprouts, which are a great protein and plant source of enzymes, vitamins and minerals. Johns Hopkins University discovered that broccoli sprouts contain up to fifty times the cancer-fighting compounds found in broccoli. They are a simple daily staple for me in summer or winter when other fresh plant food is not as available.

ONIONS, GARLIC, AND GINGER

All of these make food taste great as well as having specific beneficial health properties. Onions and garlic are considered cancer-fighting foods, especially beneficial against stomach, prostate and esophageal cancer. Onions have unique anti-inflammatory properties used to treat allergies, asthma and hay fever by blocking some of the inflammatory responses in the airways. Onions are also on the Environmental Working Group list for the top twelve foods least contaminated with pesticides.

Garlic has been used and researched for its cholesterol lowering, antithrombotic, lipid lowering, antihypertensive, antioxidant, antimicrobial, antiviral, anti-blood coagulation and antiphrastic properties. All of these benefits and more have been well documented by over twelve hundred studies. Garlic can be added to the end of cooking and is best if chopped (the finer the better). It turns out an amino acid in garlic called alliin needs to be combined with an enzyme found in garlic that is released when garlic is chopped or broken open (the finer the better). This enzyme called allinase is necessary to produce the important medical compound allicin, unique to garlic, that is responsible for its numerous health benefits.

Ginger has the ability to improve circulation, sooth an upset stomach and end nausea, making it a great remedy for morning sickness and seasickness. In studies, ginger has been shown to lower cholesterol and inhibit the oxidation of LDL cholesterol, as well as slow the development of atherosclerosis. Ginger is an antioxidant and anti-inflammatory as well.

BEANS

Beans are inexpensive, versatile and easy to cook. They are tasty, add fiber to the diet and regulate blood sugar levels. The American Institute for Cancer Research and the Nurses' Study have both shown reduced rates of cancer in men and women who consume beans as little as twice a week. Lentils are my favorite in this category. There are at least fifty types, making it easy to eat variety. Lentils also distinguish themselves from other beans because they do not contain sulphur and therefore, do not produce gas as many other types of beans have a reputation for doing. Lentils help reduce cholesterol. The soluble fiber content is high and acts as a broom as it passes through the digestive tract, clearing the way. As I mentioned, I love to sprout lentils and snack on them or toss them in my salads.

ROOT VEGETABLES

Beets, carrots and other bright orange plants (hard squashes and sweet potatoes) provide vitamin A, beta-carotene, alpha-carotene, iron and potassium. Carrots are high in carotenoids which, when consumed regularly, have been associated with decreases in colon, larynx, esophageal cancer and postmenopausal breast cancer.

Fruit

In the fruit category there are many options and I occasionally choose from them all, but I keep the daily volume of this category limited, as it is easy to fill up here and not move onto the more nutritious vegetables, nuts and seeds. I love berries as a snack, especially blueberries for their high antioxidant content. Blueberries help with fatty acid metabolism, helping to prevent plaque in the arteries as well as assisting brain function and memory. Cherries, when in season, are another good anti-inflammatory, anticancer, anti-aging snack, but only buy organic ones because they are listed by the Environmental Working Group as one of the top twelve foods contaminated by pesticides. Raspberries are another staple fruit I love to snack on. They are high in vitamin C, vitamin K, calcium, magnesium, phosphorus and fiber. Like blueberries, they are on the twelve most contaminated list and should only be bought organic. Research on raspberries has shown properties that cause the death of cancer cells and reduce the pain and inflammation of arthritis. Including fruit as a snack has proven to protect many functions of the body against dehydration to just simply keep us healthy.

I eat cranberries almost every day in a smoothie with my flax and hemp seeds. Cranberries help to keep bacteria from sticking to the lining of the urinary tract, and I love the tart taste. The last fruit on my top ten list is avocado. Its wonderful taste and the benefit of lutein, which helps the skin, eyes and heart, and keeps me eating it weekly.

Sea Vegetables

Research has shown that consuming sea vegetables may protect against environmental pollutants and radiation, which most of us do not have much control over our exposure to. They are easy to add to soups and beans and most of the time you will not even know they are there, but the benefits of consuming these sea plants is as powerful as lowering your risk of cancer. I love to snack on dried seaweed as well. All the different seaweeds contain different nutrients, but all are beneficial in their own way and worth getting to know.

Foods from these categories make a well-balanced and delicious daily addition to our diet and also help make sure we get the many vitamins, minerals, proteins, micronutrients and antioxidants we need to help build health and stay hydrated. If you would like specific nutrient values and research information on foods, check out the great book by Johnny Bowden, *The 150 Healthiest Foods on Earth: The Surprising, Unbiased Truth about What You Should Eat and Why.*

Whole Grains

Whole grains are an important part of a health supportive lifestyle. Whole grains (like rice, oats, buckwheat, millet, quinoa, wheat, spelt and oats) supply a variety of long chain complex carbohydrates, vitamins, minerals, fiber and quality oils. Balance is the key to this category of food. Do not over eat grains. They are an acid forming food if not cooked and chewed properly and we need our internal environment to remain primarily alkaline to be in optimal health.

CHAPTER 18

NATURE'S HELPING FOODS

Plants are our food and our medicine. We humans, through the processing of our food supply, have adulterated our relationship with food intended to support health and turned eating into an addiction to lifeless over-stimulating foods. Adding these foods to your diet can reverse that damage and put you back into the right relationship with what you eat.

Tomatoes protect against prostate and stomach cancer.

Tea clears clogged arteries and reduces the risk of certain cancers. *Green tea is thought to contain the highest level of polyphenols, antioxidants also found in red wine.*

Turmeric, the spice that gives curry powder its yellow color, is an antioxidant and was used as a preservative before refrigeration to keep food from going rancid.

Walnuts are cancer fighting because of their ellagic acid, it is reported that diets rich in walnuts may lower cholesterol without raising other blood triglycerides.

Carrots contain cancer-fighting compounds and protect against heart attack and stroke.

Apples help lower cholesterol.

Berries are good for vision and contain cancer-fighting compounds.

Citrus fruit helps protect against cancer.

Sesame oil and sesame seeds may prevent tumors.

Dark green leafy vegetables supply magnesium and calcium

Flaxseeds are a good source of magnesium, which helps to reduce the severity of asthma by keeping airways relaxed and open.

Flaxseeds also help lower high blood pressure and reduce the risk of heart attack and stroke in people with atherosclerosis and diabetic heart disease. They prevent the blood vessel spasm that leads to migraine attacks and generally they promote relaxation and restore normal sleep patterns.

A study published in the *Archives of Internal Medicine* confirms that eating high fiber foods, such as flaxseed, helps prevent heart disease. Almost ten thousand American adults participated in this study and were followed for nineteen years.

Flaxseed put the brakes on prostate tumor growth in men who were given thirty grams daily for a month, combined with a low-fat diet. Lead author and Duke University researcher, Wendy Demark-Wahnefried believes the Omega-3s in flaxseed alter how cancer cells lump together or cling to other cells, while flaxseed's anti-angiogenic lignans choke off the tumor's blood supply, thus helping to halt the cellular activity that leads to cancer growth.

Flaxseed meal and flour provide a very good source of fiber that, studies show, can lower cholesterol levels in people with atherosclerosis and diabetic heart disease, reduce the exposure of colon cells to cancer-causing chemicals, help relieve constipation and stabilize blood sugar levels in diabetic patients.

Flaxseed meal and flour have also been studied quite a bit lately for their beneficial, protective effects on women's health. Flaxseed is particularly rich in lignans, special compounds also found in other seeds, grains and legumes that are converted by beneficial gut flora into two hormone-like substances called enterolactone and enterodiol. These hormone-like agents demonstrate a number of protective effects against breast cancer and are believed to be one reason a vegetarian diet is associated with a lower risk of breast cancer.

Studies show that women with breast cancer and women who are omnivores typically excrete much lower levels of lignans in their urine than vegetarian women without breast cancer. In animal studies conducted to evaluate lignans' beneficial effects, supplementing a high-fat diet with flaxseed flour reduced early markers for mammary (breast) cancer in laboratory animals by more than 55 percent.

Eating about an ounce of ground flaxseed each day will affect the way estrogen is handled in postmenopausal women, in such a way that offers protection against breast cancer but will not interfere with estrogen's role in normal bone maintenance.

In addition to lessening a woman's risk of developing cancer, the lignans abundant in flaxseed can promote normal ovulation and extend the second, progesterone-dominant half of the cycle. The benefits of these effects are manifold.

For women trying to become pregnant, consistent ovulation significantly improves their chances of conception. For women between the ages of thirty-five and fifty-five who experience premenopausal symptoms, flaxseed can help reduce irregular menstrual cycles, breast cysts, headaches, sleep difficulties, fluid retention, anxiety, irritability, mood swings, weight gain, lowered sex drive, brain fog, fibroid tumors and heavy bleeding. A probable cause of all these problems is estrogen dominance.

Typically, during the ten years preceding the cessation of periods at midlife, estrogen levels fluctuate while progesterone levels steadily decline. By promoting normal ovulation and lengthening the second half of the menstrual cycle, in which progesterone is the dominant hormone, flaxseed helps restore hormonal balance.

Researchers recruited twenty-nine postmenopausal women who had suffered from at least fourteen hot flashes each week for at least one month but would not take estrogen because of a perceived increased risk of breast cancer. After taking forty grams (1.4 ounces) of crushed flaxseed each day for six weeks, the frequency of hot flashes decreased 50 percent and the overall hot flash score decreased an average 57 percent for the twenty-one women who completed the trial.

Preliminary research also suggests that flaxseeds may serve a role in protecting postmenopausal women from cardiovascular disease. In a recent double-blind randomized study, flaxseeds reduced total cholesterol levels in the blood of postmenopausal women who were not on hormone replacement therapy by an average of 6 percent.

Lastly, lignan-rich fiber has also been shown to decrease insulin resistance, which, in turn, reduces bio-available estrogen, which also lessens breast cancer risk. And, as insulin resistance is an early warning sign for type 2 diabetes, flaxseed may also provide protection against this disease.

Research indicates that for those who do not eat fish and do not wish to take fish oil supplements, flaxseed oil does provide a good alternative. A study published in the Journal of Nutrition found that flaxseed oil capsules providing three grams of alpha-linolenic acid (an amount that would be provided by three tablespoons of flaxseed oil) daily for twelve weeks increased blood levels of EPA by 60 percent in a predominantly African-American population with chronic illness. Research also shows that flaxseeds provide comparable cholesterol-lowering benefits to Statin drugs.

The INTERMAP is a study of lifestyle factors, including diet, and their effect on blood pressure in 4,680 men and women aged forty to fifty-nine, living in Japan, China, the United States and the United Kingdom. Blood pressure was measured and dietary recall questionnaires were completed by participants on four occasions. Dietary data was analyzed for levels of Omega-3 fatty acids from food sources including fish, nuts, seeds and vegetable oils. Researchers also found that Omega-3s from nuts, seeds and vegetable oils, such as walnuts and flaxseed, had just as much impact on blood pressure as Omega-3s from fish.

Flaxseed oil is especially perishable and should be purchased in opaque bottles that have been kept refrigerated. Flaxseed oil should have a sweet nutty flavor. **Never** use flaxseed oil in cooking.

CHAPTER 19

MEAL PLANNING GUIDE

I find eating simply very enjoyable and easy to maintain. If you love to cook and spend time in the kitchen, this is just the beginning. If you would rather avoid the kitchen and cooking keep it simple and eat lots of raw foods and smoothies. You will find easy fast recipes in my cookbook, *Your Health in Your Hands,* for raw food ideas and quick preparation dishes, check out katwrightnd.com.

Once you master these, you will be able to adapt any recipe for yourself or create more exotic dishes if you choose. Food should bring you pleasure, health and nourishment.

MAKING IT SIMPLE

Week one

Nutrition: start by adding a green drink first, once a day in the morning, for a week.

Fitness: take time for a twenty minute walk three days this week.

Spirit: reflect and speak about the success you have in your life.

Week two

Nutrition: add the green drink at lunch along with a fresh green mixed salad for lunch every day.

Fitness: increase your walk to five days.

Spirit: be grateful for the success in your life.

Week three

Nutrition: you are having a green drink for breakfast; now add fresh vegetable juice or cooked cereal and vegetables to your breakfast. Keep up the salad and green drink at lunch.

Fitness: increase the walk to twenty minutes twice a day for three of the days.

Spirit: tell someone else how blessed and grateful you are for the things in your life.

Week four

Nutrition: you are eating vegetables and a green drink for breakfast and lunch; now make your snacks fresh vegetables, fruits (depending on the season) and nuts.

Fitness: you are now walking forty minutes three times a week and twenty minutes twice a week; add weight-bearing exercises, such as lifting dumbbells.

Spirit: look for a group of like-minded individuals to get together with once a month or as often as it works for you, for a celebration of life and blessings.

Week five

Nutrition: you are eating vegetables and a green drink for breakfast and lunch; your snacks should be fresh vegetables, fruits (depending on the season), and nuts. Now you can start to adjust your dinners to whole nutrient-dense foods and plan your lunch by preparing leftover foods you can carry with you.

Fitness: continue the exercise and add whatever you like, such as swimming, biking, running, rebounding, or taking an aerobic class of some sort.

Spirit: tell someone about the changes you have made - invite them to join you.

Week six

Nutrition: evaluate where you are and make sure you are eating enough quality foods in general.

Fitness: make sure you are enjoying the exercise you are doing. Tell the people around you how much fun you are having.

Spirit: pick up a book or DVD that will lift you up and motivate you in a spiritual direction.

Week seven

Nutrition: look at any missing nutrients and add any needed vitamin or mineral supplements to support your activity. Remember to consider the green drink your quality vitamin and mineral supplement. If you need supplemental oils like Omega-3 or fish oil, this is a good time to add them.

Fitness: you are exercising twenty to forty minutes five days a week. Dedicate this time to you being a good steward of your body.

Spirit: ask yourself where you get your spiritual motivation and seek a mentor or accountability partner you can share with.

Week eight

Nutrition: see the following daily suggested list, you should be consuming the suggested foods and getting complete nutrition from your foods.

Fitness: start encouraging others to join you in the fitness workouts.

Spirit: celebrate that you are living a healthy lifestyle in a healthy body.

You have now supplied your body with a variety of vitamins and minerals, calcium, and mineral-rich foods, along with good quality oils, so you have a good base for a healthy, supportive lifestyle. *Your Health in Your Hands natural foods to TURN ON health and STOP disease,* will give you recipes to help you create healthy menus and delicious dishes.

You are in a healthy body and living a healthy lifestyle; share the wellness.

Breakfast

Fresh vegetable juice with flax or hemp seeds
Green drink
Two servings of fruit or vegetables

Snack

1 serving nuts or seeds
1 serving of fruit
Green drink (optional)

Lunch

1 serving of grain
2 dark green vegetables
1 yellow or orange vegetable

Snack

1 serving of nuts or seeds
1 serving of fruit
Green drink (optional)

Dinner

1 dark green leafy vegetable

1 serving of other vegetables

1 serving of protein (3-6 ounces)

Evening Snack

Tea and vegetables

Above is just an outline of a possible diet. You can eat your protein at breakfast, lunch or dinner. I discuss foods for different times of the day and you choose what sounds best to you. Remember, we make our choices based on our culture. It is not necessary to start the day with sweets, like many Americans do. Many Asians and other healthier cultures eat fish and vegetables for breakfast. Think outside of our box.

The idea here is to eat small meals, three times a day with healthy snacks in between. Be sure you are eating vegetables at every meal and have a green or fresh vegetable drink several times a day. If you eat like this, you will not be tempted to consume fast foods that were the cause of your addictions and disease in the past.

Guides for Maintaining Weight

Choose 3 – 5 small meals a day measure your snacks and keep the meals small if you choose five.

Eliminate flour products they do not digest well and cause the body to add fat.

Eliminate Refined foods they cause stress for the body and make it over work slowing metabolism.

Eliminate dairy products they are very high in sugar and cause insulin that in-turn causes extra weight gain.

Eliminate soft drinks or other beverages with high fructose corn or fruit sugars.

Natural weight loss is a result of carving out a nourishing lifestyle ...

Stop the worry, and eat only when you're relaxed. Stress hormones disrupt you body's natural functions. Measure you meals. If you do not know exactly the volume you may be overeating. Natural weight loss is a result of carving out a nourishing lifestyle with others. Finding friends and family to share life with will begin to solve the national obesity problems we have. Obesity is the beginning of all disease. Rarely does anyone succeed at tackling weight and health problems alone. Find a group of supportive individuals to start this journey with. Think for a moment who could you ask to join you? Where could you find a group to join? At the least check the web site for dates of the future *Avenues to Wellness* health and longevity retreats and workshops. www.katwrightnd.com

I celebrate and support your commitment to living well.

The Secret to your health both mind and body is not to mourn the past or worry about the future, but to live in the moment both wisely and earnestly. Anti-aging is not about looking young it is about being healthy and looking beautiful-

Kat Wright ND

Check out: **www.katwrightnd.com** for links to Free Downloadable documents

Diet Evaluation Form to measure your healthy food scores and you're aging food scores

Shopping List

This is the Beginning of your healthy life.

READING LIST AND REFERENCES

Hundreds of authors, studies, and lectures and over thirty years have gone into this work. I am listing some the best that will give you further information should you desire to read more in-depth on any of the topics I have covered. Many of the authors below have several books. I am just listing a few.

Patrick Holford: *The New Optimum Nutrition Bible*

Howard Loomis: *Enzymes: The Key to Health*

Lester Packer and Carol Colman: *The Antioxidant Miracle*

Elson M. Haas: *Staying Healthy with Nutrition*

Luise Light: *What to Eat*

J. Bowden: *The 150 Healthiest Foods on Earth: The Surprising, Unbiased Truth about What You Should Eat and Why*

Nancy Appleton: *Lick the Sugar Habit*

T. Colin Campbell and Thomas M. Campbell: *The China Study*

Paul Pitchford: *Healing with Whole Foods*

W. Wolcott and T. Fahey: *The Metabolic Typing Diet*

Michio Kushi: *The Cancer Prevention Diet*

M. Panos and J.Heimlic: *Homeopathic Medicine at Home*

www.ingramcontent.com/pod-product-compliance
Lightning Source LLC
Chambersburg PA
CBHW081351280526
45788CB00009B/2842